Living with HIV

written & edited by Michael Carter

July 2006

NAM, Lincoln House, 1 Brixton Road, London, SW9 6DE

Living with HIV
Second edition, July 2006

ISBN
1 898397 89 9

Copyright ©
NAM 2006

Production
Thomas Paterson

Illustration
Stephen Edwards

Printed in the UK by
Lithosphere, London

Thanks for the assistance of
Yusef Azad, Paul Bateman, Jackie Brown, Gus Cairns, Georgina Caswell, James Chalmers, Susan Cole, Stephen Edwards, Caroline Guinness, Dr Mark Nelson, Will Nutland, Carolyn Partrick, Nick Partridge, Roger Pebody, Chris Smith, Positive Nation, Positively Women, all my colleagues at NAM, and everybody who took the time and effort to write about their lives with HIV

NAM contact details

NAM, Lincoln House, 1 Brixton Road, London, SW9 6DE, UK
email: info@nam.org.uk   tel: 020 7840 0050   fax: 020 7735 5351   website: www.aidsmap.com

NAM — for HIV information

NAM was founded by Peter Scott in 1987. He was working at the heart of the community affected by HIV - at the London Lesbian and Gay Switchboard. At that time it was important to produce a clear, plain language resource in the face of extensive misinformation about HIV and AIDS, much of it confused and homophobic.

NAM now also publishes a wide range of printed, audio and electronic materials for all communities of people with HIV and publishes on the internet at www.aidsmap.com. The work is rooted in the experiences of those most affected by the epidemic.

NAM believes information enables people to take control of their lives and healthcare, develop better dialogues with their healthcare staff and so live longer, healthier lives.

Preface to the Second Edition

When I was first diagnosed with HIV, eighteen years ago, we knew virtually nothing about what this virus was, how it worked, or how to stop it causing havoc in our immune systems. There was no treatment, precious little knowledge, and widespread prejudice and fear. We all assumed that life expectancy would be short.

A huge amount has changed since then. Scientific understanding has grown in leaps and bounds. Public knowledge has certainly improved, though some prejudice still lingers. The development of powerful combinations of anti-HIV drugs (such as the ones I take) has transformed the nature and prospects of treatment. There are now eighteen drugs licensed, with more in development, and for those newly diagnosed with HIV or doing well on anti-HIV therapy the prognosis is infinitely better than it was.

Yet many things have remained unchanged. Having HIV and taking combination therapy isn't easy, and side-effects are sometimes hard. You still need to look after your health generally. We have to continue to stand up to intolerance and ignorance. And the support of partners, friends and colleagues is as important today as it was eighteen years ago.

In 1988, information - however sketchy - was the key to understanding what being HIV-positive meant. Information is still the key today. And this book - with its accompanying first-hand accounts of the reality of life with HIV - provides an excellent introduction to the issues which so many of us affected by HIV live with, day-by-day. It is packed with information; and for those affected by HIV - be they living with the virus, connected with or caring for those who are, or simply interested and concerned - it is of real value.

Chris Smith
Rt Hon Lord Smith of Finsbury

Preface to the First Edition

The first guide to survival written by people living with AIDS in the UK was published in 1987. Looking at "Living with AIDS" now and comparing it to "Living with HIV 2004" shows both how much has changed and how much we still have in common with those writing 17 years ago.

Many of the personal issues remain - coming to terms with your diagnosis, who to tell, looking after yourself, sex life, employment, coping with fear, illness and going into hospital. But the emphasis is wholly different. In 1987, preparing for the future included making a will and considering the kind of funeral you would want. Now, for many people, it's about staying in work and planning for a pension.

"Living with AIDS" was just 20 pages long, mentioned only two anti-HIV drugs and yet was optimistic about research and the future. For many, that optimistic future has arrived. So we now need to understand things like viral load and CD4 counts, combinations of 18 drugs in four classes with more to come - as well as getting on with life.

Like its predecessors, this book comes directly from the experience of people living with HIV. It pools and shares information, knowledge and insight, which has always been the foundation for taking control of any illness. For anyone living with HIV, this guide will be invaluable.

Nick Partridge OBE
Chief Executive, Terrence Higgins Trust

Contents

Living with HIV   **2**
Introduction 4

Just found out you're HIV-positive?   **16**
Finding out the basics 18
Getting HIV treatment and care 19
Finding out about tests 19
Making decisions 19
You're not alone 21

HIV, the basics   **30**
HIV 32
AIDS 32
HIV transmission 32
The HIV test 33
Stages of HIV infection 33
HIV treatments - the changed reality of living with HIV 35

Telling people you are HIV-positive   **42**
Don't rush 44
Practicalities 44
Telling your partner 45
Telling sexual partners 45
Telling ex-partners 45
Family 46
Friends 46
Work 46
Healthcare professionals 47
Children 49

Getting HIV treatment and care   **56**
HIV clinics 58
You and your doctor 60
GPs 61
Dentists 64
NHS care and non-UK nationals 64

Key tests to monitor HIV- CD4 and viral load   72

Why monitor? 74
CD4 cell counts 74
Viral load 78
Looking at CD4 and viral load together 80
Frequency of testing 82
Other tests 82

Anti-HIV treatment   86

Treatment, not a cure 88
When to start treatment 88
Starting anti-HIV treatment 91
Anti-HIV drug classes and names 91
First combination 92
Which nucleotides/nucleotide? 93
Questions to ask your doctor before starting treatment 95
Changing treatment due to failure 101
Changing treatment due to side-effects 102
Changing treatment due to lipodystrophy 102
Salvage therapy 103
Treatment breaks 105

Adherence - taking your medicine   116

Why adherence is important 118
Level of adherence to aim for 119
How to boost your chances of adherence 120
Late doses 121
Support from your clinic 122
Adherence tips 123

Side-effects   128

Types of side-effects 130
When side-effects develop 131
Coping with side-effects 132
Nausea, lipodystrophy and peripheral neuropathy 132
Nausea and vomiting 133
Lipodystrophy 134
Peripheral neuropathy 142

Symptoms and illnesses   154

Symptoms 156
Illnesses 160
Illnesses in the age of anti-HIV treatment - cancers .165
Illnesses in the age of anti-HIV treatment - hepatitis 167

Mother-to-baby transmission of HIV   186

Preventing mother-to-baby transmission with anti-HIV drugs 188
Safety of treatment to prevent mother-to-baby transmission of HIV 190
Preventing mother-to-baby transmission of HIV 190

Complementary therapies   196
Reasons why people with HIV use complementary therapies 198
Points to remember 199
Choosing a therapist 199
Combining conventional and complementary therapies 200
A-Z of complementary therapies 201

Daily health issues   208
Day-to-day hygiene 210
Pets and animals 210
Drinking water 211
Food poisoning 214
International travel 215
Vaccinations and immunisations 216
Sex 216
Recreational drug use 219
Safer drug use 235

Coping with illness, going into hospital, end of life issues   240
Coping with illness 242
Going into hospital 243
End of life issues 247

Nutrition and HIV   256
A good diet 258
Dietitians 258
Supplements 259
Alcohol in diet 260
Food, drink and anti-HIV drugs 260
Lipodystrophy and diet 261
Weight loss 261
Diarrhoea and diet 261

Exercise   264
Benefits of exercise 266
Planning for exercise 266
Types of exercise 267
Sustaining exercise 268
Fuel for exercise 268
Steroids 269

Mental health   272
HIV-related mental disorders 274
Emotional distress 275
Depression 276
Mental health problems as a side-effect of anti-HIV treatment 277
Anxiety 277
Talking therapies 278

Sex   288

HIV sex and you 290
Dealing with sexual problems 291
HIV sex and the law 293
Sexual health 293
Sexual health check-ups 293
Protecting your own and other people's sexual health 294
Use of anti-HIV drugs to prevent infection with HIV 296
Undetectable viral load and infectiousness 297
Reinfection 297

Money   308

State benefits 310
The Regulated Social Fund 321
Personal finance 322

Travel   324

Introduction 326
Entry restrictions 326
Countries and their entry restrictions 327
Problems getting into the UK 337
Travelling with medication 338
In good enough health to travel? 339
Travel insurance 339
Reciprocal medical care 339
Vaccinations 340
Treatment breaks and travel 340

Work   344

Going back to work 346
Working with HIV 348

HIV and the law, by James Chalmers   350

Confidentiality 352
HIV transmission and the criminal law 355
Immigration and asylum law 357
Disability Discrimination Act (DDA) 360

Finding information   366

National Helplines 368
Key self-help, advocacy and specialist groups 369
Websites 371

Index   375

Personal Stories

Life on HIV treatment, a personal perspective by Michael Carter 6

My life with HIV, by Maureen 10

An emotional rollercoaster, by Winnie Ssanyu Sseruma 12

Time will tell, by Paul 22

Rob 23

Lorraine's story 24

February 12th, 2005 26

Pamella 27

The bus of doom, by Caroline Guinness 38

20 years and counting 40

Grateful? I don't think so, by Susan 50

Telling people, by Alan 51

Anciciaria's story 68

First refusal, by Alan 107

Starting treatment, by Christopher 108

Finally undetectable!, by Edwin 110

Robert and treatment 112

From devastation to optimism 113

Jewelled friends, by Alan 126

New life, *New Fill*, by Edwin 145

Chris's peripheral neuropathy 146

Michael, what he did about his peripheral neuropathy .147

It's all arse over face, by Myles 148

Headaches, by Martin 174

It's the bigots I feel sorry for 175

No bed of roses 177

TB - my experiences, by Nick 178

Paul, living with HIV and hepatitis C and haemophilia 180

The luxury of hypochondriacs, by Caroline Guinness 183

Matilda 192

Bun in the oven 193

The Ikea approach .... .205

Billy .... .250

Going into hospital, by Christopher .... .253

Ironman .... .270

A permanent feature .... .279

Alone, by John .... .282

Coping, by Frank .... .283

Russ .... .284

My experience of anal warts .... .299

My hero!, by Philip .... .301

Bored and horny .... .303

Holiday hassles and HRT, by Caroline Guinness .... .341

Anger .... .362

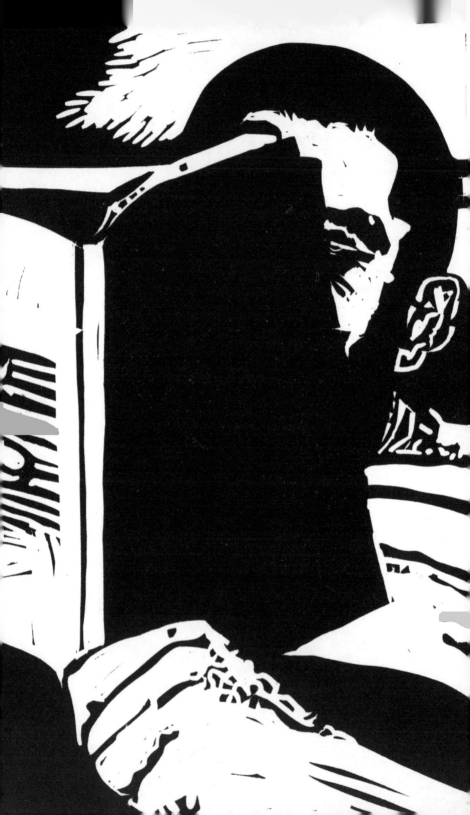

Introduction

Living with HIV

In this chapter you'll find

An explanation of who this book is for.

A summary of previous editions of this book
and an acknowledgement of the help of
those who helped in its preparation.

Three first hand testimonies of life with
HIV, one from an HIV-positive gay man and
two from African women.

This book is for people who are HIV-positive. It's hoped that it will contain something useful both for people who have been recently diagnosed with HIV and for those who have known that they have HIV for some time. It's been written with a UK readership in mind.

The book includes information on the medical and social aspects of life with HIV and aims to provide basic answers to some of the questions you may find yourself asking. You might want to read the book cover-to-cover, or just dip into it at times when you need to find something out.

The information in this book isn't exhaustive, and it isn't intended to replace discussions with your doctor or any other professional. But it should provide an introduction to the key issues involved in living with HIV and help you decide what further questions you may need to ask.

NAM produces a range of HIV information books, booklets and leaflets, and some of these are listed (along with publications from THT and the UK Coalition of People Living with HIV and AIDS) at the end of each chapter as suggestions for further reading.

Included in the book are first-hand accounts written by people who are living with HIV. They're not meant to be examples of what you should do, they just give an idea of how people have coped with the realities of day-to-day life with HIV. Thanks to everybody who sent contributions. Every effort was made to include them all, but there simply wasn't room. Sorry if yours wasn't included.

This is the second edition of *Living with HIV*. The information contained in the first edition has been updated and the chapters on sex, money, and HIV and the law have been thoroughly revised.

Living with HIV has a history dating back almost 20 years and is a direct successor to *Living with HIV and AIDS*, published by NAM in early 1996 and the 1987 Frontliners' publication, *Living with AIDS*. This edition of *Living with HIV* (and the 2004 first edition), reflects the tremendous advances made in HIV treatment since the mid-1990s, but also acknowledges the real problems that life with HIV can involve.

Information from NAM's *HIV and AIDS Reference Manual* has been adapted for inclusion in this book.

Thanks to everybody who was involved in the preparation of *Living with HIV and AIDS* and editions of the *HIV and AIDS Reference Manual*. Your hard work has made the preparation of this book a lot easier than it would otherwise have been.

I'd also like to record my thanks to Chris Smith for providing the preface to this edition, Jackie Brown, formerly of THT, for contributing the section on state benefits, James Chalmers for contributing a chapter on HIV and the law, and Steve Edwards for his enthusiastic and tireless work illustrating this book.

There are three of us in our relationship – Paul, HIV and me. Paul is the most important, he cooks the tea.

positive voice

Life on HIV treatment
a personal perspective by Michael Carter

I've been taking antiretroviral therapy for the last eight years. I've seen my CD4 cell count quadruple and my viral load fall from the high hundred thousands to below 50 and stay there. It would be easy to conclude that, for me, the treatments have been a success - not least because it's over 15 years since I was diagnosed with HIV and 13 years since my first AIDS-defining illness. To put it simply, without anti-HIV drugs I expect I would be dead now. Instead, I'm alive and in excellent health.

However, I am still very much aware of the seriousness of HIV, of the extent to which it affects my life and of the fact that it is likely to continue to do so for the foreseeable future.

First of all, I still get ill because of HIV. In early 2005 I developed a high fever and cough. My temperature quickly returned to normal, but my cough stayed put. Six months later my temperature dramatically returned resulting in my hospitalisation whilst attending a conference in Spain. A chest X-ray revealed that I had pneumonia, and further tests on my return to the UK identified a multi-drug resistant pneumonia bug. Over a year later, despite having a CD4 cell count in the high hundreds, the bug is still present, and still makes me cough. My consultant is in no doubt that the reason I have it is because I'm HIV-positive.

What's more, I'm still very medicalised. I go to the HIV clinic every twelve weeks for blood tests to monitor the success of my treatment and its impact on my metabolism. This means that I see my consultant just as often as I did before I started taking anti-HIV drugs.

Living with HIV has also had an impact on my mental health - just as the lab results began to suggest that the damage it was doing to my immune system was being controlled, my mental health declined. I've had two major depressions since I started HIV treatment, each of them as debilitating in their own way as any physical illness HIV has caused me. Both my consultant and the specialist HIV psychiatrist he referred me to have assured me that I'm far from alone in experiencing mental health problems after starting treatment. For some, these are direct side-effects of their medication. For me, the causes have been less direct. I've had periods of real pessimism, and the renewed hope for the future which treatment has given me has been compromised by side-effects and uncertainty.

Fortunately, I've been spared any of the disfiguring changes in body shape (lipodystrophy) which some anti-HIV treatments can cause. A friend, however, has not been so lucky, and has developed severe facial wasting which has required several courses of treatment to correct even temporarily. As he put it: "It's the ultimate irony - you're spared dying of AIDS only to look as if you are".

I've had my fair share of side-effects as well, including the diarrhoea that accompanied my first year on nelfinavir, which felt like a tap being turned on in my bowels. Then there was the peripheral neuropathy in my feet and lower legs - the worst pain I've ever been in, which still isn't completely resolved, five years after stopping the drug which caused it. At one point I had to see a cardiologist, after I developed an irregular heart beat. As I've no obvious risk factors for heart disease - indeed, I've run several marathons - the increased blood fats which some anti-HIV drugs can cause looked like a possible cause. Thankfully it turned out to be nothing more worrying than the consequence of having a low resting heart rate, from all the running I do. But it required numerous visits to the hospital, and I still ask my doctor about my cholesterol levels with some concern.

When I'm feeling optimistic, I can well envisage anti-HIV treatment keeping me well and living to a ripe old age. But every time I have my viral load measured, I worry that it may have become detectable again. I'm only human, and despite my best efforts I occasionally miss taking a dose of my treatment or take it a few hours late.

I'm also uncertain about how long my body can tolerate infection with a chronic viral illness like HIV and the potent drugs needed to treat it. I'm more than aware of the excess rates of certain cancers seen in people with HIV, and, as I've had warts in my anus and rectum in the past, I'm particularly concerned by reports that even when anti-HIV drugs are working well, people with HIV who've had anal warts have an increased risk of anal cancer.

Coupled with the medical uncertainty is a lack of security, particularly regarding money. Although I've managed to stay in the same job for over four years now, HIV meant that I had a very chequered employment history for over a decade. I'm now fast approaching 40, and don't own my own home (and doubt that I ever will). I've started paying into a personal pension plan, but worry that I've left it too late. I really do worry that chronic poverty could be awaiting me in old age - if HIV treatment keeps me alive that long.

But there's a need for a bit of perspective. I'm not the only person I know who worries about money and security. It's far too easy to blame HIV and treatment side-effects for just about every medical condition that raises its head. For example, I noticed a slight thinning in my cheeks recently, and my instincts were to attribute this to treatment-associated fat loss rather than to look at a less sinister explanation, like the fact that I'm getting older.

With treatment has also come a redefinition in the way I perceive myself and, I think, the way others look at me. I've no doubt that I'll live a longer and healthier life thanks to antiretroviral therapy. This means I'm starting to expect things from life - not least enjoyment and fulfilment. I'm no longer prepared to accept the day-to-day drudge that accompanied my pre-treatment days with HIV. Nor, if another drug option exists, do I see why I should have to cope with side-effects. I've become bored of hiding my HIV status - if somebody asks me how I got a housing association flat with a garden in central London I now tell them, "because I have AIDS." It normally stops any further questioning. Nor do I worry about looks or enquiries when I take my pills in public.

But there are still limitations to my honesty and openness. I've never told my parents I have HIV. This isn't because I fear that they will reject me; on the contrary I know that they love me unconditionally; but I wonder how much good it would do them or me - would it be just another source of worry for them in their old age?

I'm lucky that I've never had a bad reaction from anyone I've told I was HIV-positive - yet.

But despite my best efforts, popular prejudice about HIV has penetrated deep into my consciousness. I do feel guilty that the medical services provided for my treatment are so good when my chronically ill parents have to wait months for appointments and even longer for treatment and care. And uncomfortable as it is to admit this, I do sometimes wonder that the reason why I never told them was a legacy of the internalised homophobia I struggled with for much of my adult life and a deep seated shame about becoming HIV-positive in the first place. This hasn't been helped at all by the recent criminalisation of HIV transmission in the UK.

Thanks to the success of treatment, I no longer feel that people should make the allowances for me that they were prepared to make in the past. I'm very aware of how hard it's been for my partner and friends at times. The problems I'm facing now are less serious, and are more generic - a lot of people have controllable chronic illnesses; a lot of people live with pain; a lot of people are financially insecure.

I want to make the most of the fact that HIV treatment means that I'm alive and planning for the future when I expected to be dead. But I also need to acknowledge that life with HIV medication brings its own set of problems. Like HIV itself, they've become part of my life, and, with varying degrees of success, I've had to find ways of coping with them.

My life with HIV
by Maureen

I was born in Zambia 1973 and came to England in April 1994 to live with my cousin to help her look after her three children. Soon after, I had swollen legs and I went to accident and emergency where I was told I had an acute febrile illness. I was admitted to Queen Mary's University Hospital Roehampton. In July 1994 I was asked if they could do a HIV test and I agreed. I didn't know anything about HIV. Back in Zambia the word HIV was unspoken. I had heard of AIDS which I only associated with death. Three days later I was diagnosed HIV-positive. I was 19 years old when they told me and explained that I was HIV-positive. I was shocked, upset and I couldn't speak to anyone. Later that day I asked myself why, why me?

When I was told, my auntie and my cousin's husband were standing there and I could hear them say in my language 'She has to go back home. Who is going look after her? Who will tell her that we can't look after her?'

I just wanted someone to say to me that everything will be alright but no one did. The pain I felt in my heart grew stronger and the feeling I had, I knew, wasn't good. I was lost and confused. No one asked me what I wanted. I needed my mother and father to be there. I started crying. I waited. I agonised with the thought of going back home with this family whom I could see didn't want me there. To them I was a dead person walking.

I started worrying. When 'my time' came would I have anyone to sit at my bedside with me? Another worry was that being the first born in my family meant I was expected to provide for them. How was I going to tell my mummy, daddy, brothers and sisters when I go back to Zambia? Yet it became important to me to accept the situation that I am HIV-positive. I needed to be strong for my family and myself. Again, I kept asking myself why me?

Finally, my aunt made the decision that I would go back and live with them. This was on the condition that I would not talk about my illness nor my feelings. At the same time the children would have returned to school.

I started seeing my consultant and a health advisor at a clinic in south west London. At first, appointments were weekly then monthly. My CD4 count was 460. In January 1997 my viral load was tested for the first time and it was 750,000. I was told that such a high level suggested I was at risk of becoming ill because of HIV in the near future. In February 1997 my doctor from the clinic phoned to say and asked me to come in and see him. I asked why, and was told it was time to start taking anti-HIV drugs. I remember falling down on the floor with the phone in my hand. As I was having lunch with my cousin and the children, my cousin took the phone from me and started talking to my doctor. The silence, sadness, everything came back again and the things I wanted to stay in the past started to invade my thoughts and were here again with me in the future.

The thought of taking the medication everyday of my life was like the feeling of drowning. I felt the pain coming back again and I was in shock.

Later I gave myself a good talking to, and made the decision to accept and start taking the medication. Unfortunately, I started having side-effects, feeling tired all the time but worst of all I couldn't tell anyone how I was feeling. I kept waiting for someone to talk to, but the pain inside me was growing everyday.

Living with HIV changed everything in my life. In late 1997 I moved to central London and registered at a new HIV clinic. In 2000 I developed resistance to the drugs I was taking. I had a break from the drugs between November 2000 and November 2002. Then I started taking different medication and again started to have side-effects. I was feeling tired, dizzy, with diarrhoea and nausea. I changed the drugs again. I had a different set of side-effects. My stomach grew and I looked like I was pregnant. I didn't like it. Once when I was on the bus someone offered me a seat and said "in your condition you shouldn't be standing, have a seat". I was upset and looking at this person I said "no thank you, I am not pregnant". Everyone looked at me. I could feel what they were thinking and saying in their hearts. After that the feeling

I had wasn't good and I started crying. I felt pain, hate and anger every time I thought about HIV.

Now I know I am not alone. I have support from other people and I give support to others as well. I think living with HIV has made me stronger and I believe that once I accepted it and learnt to move on, life became easier. But I have to say I wouldn't wish this on anyone in the world. I think being HIV-positive made me not want to be in a relationship with anyone, but yes, I would like to find someone who will accept me for who I am.

An emotional rollercoaster
by Winnie Ssanyu Sseruma

If someone would have told me that I would be alive 18 years after my HIV diagnosis I would not have believed them. As I write I am two days away from my 45th birthday, far older that most people in African countries now expect to live.

I could never have imagined my life after my HIV diagnosis, but it continues to amaze me. Unlike many people living with HIV, I do not particularly remember the day I was diagnosed (maybe I blocked it out), but I just know that what I totally underestimated is the emotional roller coaster HIV set me on.

The first six years of my diagnosis were the absolute worst, I just didn't know whether to carry on or to give up on life from one day to the next. Apart from worrying about my health there was so much else going on with my family that it was hard to concentrate on myself. I was living in the US on my own and my whole family was a long way away in Uganda. I lost a brother to HIV and both my parents died from different forms of cancer never knowing about my status. I feel it was a blessing in disguise for me because at the time, I didn't feel it was an option for me to tell them.

When I left the US to go back to Uganda in 1994 it was simply to die because I was mentally and physically exhausted and could not see a way forward. I was so depressed and utterly desperate, but received no official diagnosis for my depression. After six months in Uganda, I fell ill with tuberculosis, PCP and diarrhoea and almost got my wish of dying. However, for someone who wanted to die, I quickly went to the doctor with the onset of symptoms of any opportunistic infection, was very clear in terms of explaining the symptoms and was able to pay for my treatment. I believe that it was because of those specific steps that I took that I am partly alive now.

In 1996, I moved to live in the UK for the first time, even though that is where I was born. My mental state was still very fragile and I was not sure whether I wanted to start a new life or let nature take its course. Moving to the UK energised me as I saw, met and spoke to people living with HIV for the first time. I started accessing services including support groups, counselling and anti-HIV treatment. My health stabilised which left me with enough energy to want to live again.

Ten years on, I have never felt better about myself. The biggest challenge I face is pacing myself. I usually fail miserably. Many times I forget I am living with the virus even when I have to take my medication. There are a number of things that have helped me focus on living a full life again, apart from those that I have already mentioned. Remaining active with work, constantly networking and travelling have all kept me quite sane. I do not have time to feel sorry for myself. Being openly positive and knowing that I do not have to hide my status from anyone has been incredibly liberating. The wisdom that comes with age, feeling comfortable about oneself and not worrying about what anyone else thinks has had a huge impact on my life.

I have never looked back to ask questions like why me, I am totally at ease with myself. It is an amazing feeling given what many people think living with HIV is or ought to be.

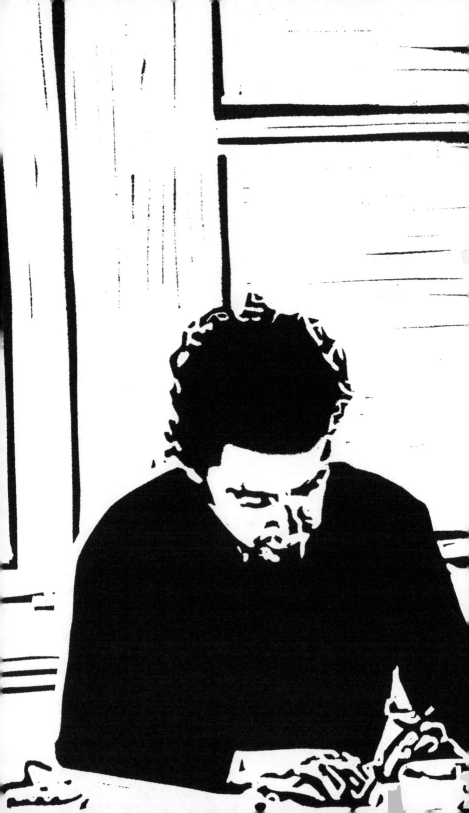

Just found out you're HIV-positive?

In this chapter you'll find information on

Why it's important to know that you have HIV.

Some commonly asked questions following an HIV diagnosis.

Details of how to get HIV treatment and care.

Some basic information on key tests to monitor HIV.

Details of THT Direct and the National Sexual Health Helpline.

Five people - two women, a heterosexual man and two gay men contributed testimonies about finding out they had HIV.

Introduction

Being diagnosed with HIV will be one of the most significant events in your life. It's very difficult to predict exactly what emotions and feelings you'll experience in the first few hours and days after finding out you have HIV, as these vary so widely from individual to individual. However, commonly reported reactions include feeling numb, frightened, upset, tearful, desperate or angry. Although it should be noted that other people have said they were relieved to have finally found out, or even excited.

It might be difficult to appreciate this at the time, but finding out that you are HIV-positive puts you in a position where you can start to take steps towards looking after your health. Although there's no cure for HIV and it can still be fatal, there are treatments which mean that people with HIV can live much longer and healthier lives. The sooner your HIV infection is diagnosed, the sooner you can receive appropriate medical care.

The fact that you have HIV might be the only information you can absorb on the day of your diagnosis. You should have had post-test counselling after you received your test result, and you may have been able to ask a few questions at this stage. There are no right or wrong questions to ask, and don't worry if you didn't understand everything you were told. There'll be opportunities to get more information later.

Finding out the basics

It's perfectly okay to want the most basic information, such as, "What's the difference between HIV and AIDS?" Or, "How long before HIV makes me ill?' Or, 'Will HIV kill me?" The first chapter of this book, "HIV, the basics", should answer your questions.

You may also come across lots of medical terms you don't understand. Always ask your doctor, a nurse or a pharmacist to explain anything you don't understand, and ask for written information if you still have questions or uncertainties. If you want more detailed information on a particular topic, the chances are that there'll be a chapter in this book focusing on the subject you're interested in.

Getting HIV treatment and care

You are going to need specialist medical care for your HIV. Most people in this country are tested for HIV at sexual health clinics (although some people are diagnosed through other medical services), which usually have a specialist HIV clinic attached. The doctor, nurse or counsellor who gave you your test result should have made a follow-up appointment for you to see a specialist HIV doctor. If this wasn't arranged, you need to make sure that you are registered with a specialist HIV clinic as soon as possible. There's information on this in the chapter *Getting HIV treatment and care.*

If you are well at the time of your HIV diagnosis, you'll probably need to go to the clinic for a check-up every three months or so. At your appointment with your doctor you'll have an opportunity to discuss your health and ask questions, and you will have some blood tests to monitor your health.

Finding out about tests

There are two key blood tests used to assess the impact HIV is having on your immune system. These are called CD4 cell counts and viral load tests. A CD4 cell count gives a rough idea of how healthy your immune system is, and the viral load test gives an indication of how active HIV is in your body. The more active HIV is, the lower your CD4 cell count becomes, and the greater your risk of becoming unwell because of HIV. Find out more about these tests by reading the chapter *Key tests to monitor HIV.*

Making decisions

Immediately after your diagnosis can be a difficult time to make major decisions. These decisions might include who to tell about your HIV diagnosis or when to start anti-HIV treatment.

It's highly unlikely that you are asked to start taking anti-HIV treatment the day you found out that you were HIV-positive. It's more likely that your health will be monitored, so both you and your doctor can understand how your body is coping with HIV. If your immune system has already been weakened by HIV, then the decision to start taking anti-HIV drugs to prevent you getting the infections and illnesses to which HIV can make you vulnerable will be a more pressing one. But anti-HIV treatment is something that you will need to consider sooner or later. In this book you can find out when you need to start treatment, what medicines you need to take, how often you need to take your medicines and what side-effects you might experience.

Take time to think about who you are going to tell that you are HIV-positive. Think about why you want to tell them and how you are going to tell them. Can you anticipate their best or worst reactions? Begin by telling the people closest to you, who will be the most supportive. This book includes a chapter, *Telling people you are HIV-positive* which provides more information on telling people in all sorts of situations.

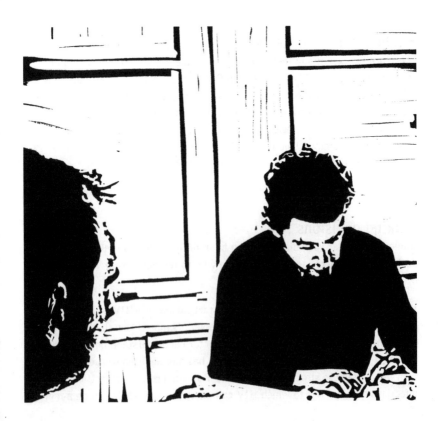

You're not alone

A lot of professional support is available to you. In the weeks and months after your diagnosis, you might find that counselling helps you work out your reactions to having HIV.

There are two helplines which you might find particularly useful at this time, both of which can provide basic information on HIV and are staffed by trained counsellors who will help you talk through some of your feelings.

These helplines are:

- THT Direct on 0845 122 1200.
- National Sexual Health Helpline on 0800 567 123

Knowing that you're not the only person going through your experiences might also be helpful, and some people find that meeting other HIV-positive people helps them to overcome their own feelings of stigma about having HIV. Some HIV organisations have events for the recently diagnosed. Don't feel that you have to attend a group if you're not comfortable with the idea, and don't think you've made a mistake if you've reacted to your diagnosis differently than somebody else has. There's no right or wrong way to respond to finding out you have HIV - the important thing is that you start to get information and medical care so that you can stay healthy and live as long as possible.

This book should provide a useful first step.

Further reading

- *10 Things it's good to know about HIV*, NAM leaflet.
- NAM factsheet, *Recently diagnosed*.
- 'Introduction to HIV and AIDS,' in NAM's *HIV and AIDS Treatment Directory*.
- *What now?*, booklet produced by the Terrence Higgins Trust.
- *Tell me about HIV*, booklet produced by the UK Coalition of People Living with HIV and AIDS.

Time will tell
by Paul

I was devastated when I got the news that I was HIV-positive. But I was lucky to have such a supportive GP. It was thanks to her that I had an HIV test in the first place - I had a wart on my face that she thought looked a bit funny and recommended that I go for a test. It came back positive on 29th March 2005. My GP made me the appointment at the GUM clinic in Edinburgh for the 31st March and the staff were so helpful and friendly. I got my bloods taken and I started to get counselling. I was told that, looking at my CD4 cell count and viral load, to expect to be on treatment within a year.

I started the treatment on 18th August 2005. I was ill for the first week and was vomiting morning and night before meals but I stuck it out. I got my bloods done a month after being on treatment. My viral load went from 198,000 to 1,840 and CD4 cell count from 244 to 304. I started to feel much better as the weeks went by and have never missed my doses, which I take twice a day at 7.30am and 7.30pm. Military precision!

My work was a different matter. At first I was supported and then a woman claimed I forced knowledge of my diagnosis onto her and caused trouble. I was taken in by my manager and personnel and was treated like a school child. I had to take ten weeks off work and let everything settle. They never called me once to see how I was getting on. I went back to work and was very wary of all the managers and that dreadful woman.

I do my job but find I get tired and stressed now, so I am thinking of looking for another job.

My mother, sister and her partner have been fantastic about my diagnosis and my close friends too.

I feel that I cannot go out and meet a potential partner as I'm scared of the reaction when they find out what I have and how I would feel if I was rejected again.

I still see a psychologist which has helped me immensely over the past seven months and my consultant has been a big help too.

I hope as the weeks go on that I will improve, but time will tell.

Rob

I was given my diagnosis over the telephone after spending four days in hospital with meningitis. I now realise it wasn't meningitis, it was an HIV seroconversion illness. I literally couldn't get out of bed one day and ended up in A&E. I was terrified and alone and I asked if it could be HIV. The ward was overcrowded and no one saw me for three days after an initial consultation except the nurse who told me nothing. Then I was discharged.

I don't know why, but I knew that couldn't be the end of it. I went for an antigen test.

After the initial shock of being told that I had HIV over the phone by a doctor, I was in a daze for about a week. I didn't know where to go or what to do. I just sat there most days, not knowing how to go on and wanting to hit out because it was so unfair; it's not fair for anyone.

After being told I would have to be retested before I could get a place in a clinic, I nearly broke down, I knew I was positive and didn't want to go through more tests.

Then I got to speak to an amazing senior health worker and things started to change. I left with an appointment to see a consultant and a smile for the first time in weeks.

My blood results were erratic as to be expected and I'm still waiting for them to stabilise, fingers crossed, but I knew all that and I expected it. What I hadn't expected was the anxiety and panic attacks, the nightmares I had and the lack of breath. It took a while for me to calm down about it and I am not usually an anxious person. These were totally new experiences to me and I was finding it tough. Combined with the dermatitis, fatigue and continual stomach bugs I experienced, I felt like I was falling apart.

I'm not saying all this to cause worry; I'm saying all this because if I'd have known to expect some of this, it wouldn't have been so hard. Jumping hurdles is easier if you can see them.

It's been seven months now and for the first time I'm actually feeling okay about it. Obviously I still worry about things, particular the future, I never felt so mortal before and my long-term health still concerns me, but I feel ok.

I feel OK because I feel like I know what to expect now. I have a different outlook on things. I feel better for knowing my status and I'm making so much more of my life than I was before. I think about where I'll be in 15 years, not in a bad way, in a good way, I want to have done something.

Lorraine's story

I was diagnosed HIV-positive five and a half years ago. My husband had been ill for the previous 18 months, but not with anything they could put a name to. It was only when he went into hospital for tests to find out why he was literally wasting away that they found out he had pneumonia. More tests revealed it was PCP.

The night he told me that he was HIV-positive, I was relieved, which was a funny reaction. I thought that at least we had a name to his illness and he could be treated. Later on, I thought about myself and whether I was infected. We were both under the impression that I would be fine, as I looked and felt really healthy. But then the GP rang me the next night...

The following weeks passed in a daze. My husband developed an infection, which, combined with working and looking after our two children, meant nothing sank in.

I knew nothing about HIV, but not through complacency - I had seen the government advertising campaigns in the late 1980s, but I had been married for 18 years. Now, I had so many questions, so many fears. The emotions I experienced were so complex I couldn't put them into words. I could just about cope from minute to minute.

Meanwhile, my husband made a partial recovery but was given only weeks to live. I left my work to focus on keeping the family together for however long we had. A few months later, things had sunk in, and I contacted the George House Trust in Manchester. There I met the most wonderful, inspiring group of women. With their support, strength and experiences, I began to feel human again. Unfortunately, my husband died the following year. A few months later, combination therapy became available and suddenly there was hope.

When I was first diagnosed, the only thing I wanted was to speak to another woman who had gone through the same thing. So when I saw the position for regional coordinator advertised, I applied. I thought that if I could be of help to anyone I would, in a way, be giving back all the support I had received.

We have a very good support group in Manchester, and doing my voluntary work has made me realise how lucky I was to have that support. There are many women around the country who are isolated - through fear of being 'found out', through not knowing who to contact, because they are carers or mothers or because they have no transport or facilities nearby. That is why this work is important - I can be just a voice on the telephone, a point of contact as and when it is required or I can arrange to meet up with them, one to one. Then perhaps, when they are ready, I can introduce them to local support services. Everyone is different and their circumstances and needs change, but no one should go through it alone.

This testimony first appeared on the website of Positively Women, www.positivelywomen.org.uk. Thanks to both the writer and Positively Women for giving permission to reprint it here.

February 12th, 2005

I was diagnosed HIV-positive on February 12th 2005 - two days after splitting up with my wife of nine years. I was shocked at first, but came to accept it - I knew the risks of unprotected sex and I had had a fling with another man the year before.

My main - and very major concern - was having to reveal my status to my wife and worry as to whether she and our young kids had been infected with HIV. After a harrowing two months they got the all clear and my wife was actually really supportive to me.

I think the disease has given me a better perspective on life. I'm clearer about my priorities and what's really important to me. I'm slightly more selfish than I used to be - not unreasonably so - but I'm determined to do what I want to do and not continue running around after everyone else's demands. I'm not yet back with my wife - I live in rented accommodation and don't want to get back into the relationship unless I'm sure it can work again. That's also part of my 'reduce stress' self-defence.

I've found the people at my specialist HIV clinic and THT really supportive (I did twelve sessions of counselling last summer with THT to try to get to the bottom of my feelings, particularly about life and relationships) which turned out, even though I was initially very cynical, to be really useful. I've also found other people with HIV a great source of inspiration, support and advice.

I remain optimistic about the future and look forward to spending much more time with my kids.

Pamella

I found out I had HIV in June 2005. My world just fell apart. I didn't know that I needed an HIV test, but the nurse at my GP suggested that I should go to a GUM clinic and have one because I had thrush.

Well, I didn't know what a GUM clinic was and when I found it at my local hospital I panicked when I saw the posters about HIV and sexually transmitted infections. But then I told myself to calm down as I had been through similar experiences before. The year before I was diagnosed with a brain tumour and had a lot of tests, although I wasn't tested for HIV.

Two weeks later I went back to the hospital to get my results. The health advisor told me I had HIV and that my CD4 cell count was 72. I didn't know what that meant.

Believe me, I can't describe the emotions that were flowing within me. I felt that my whole life had been snatched away from me. All my plans dissolved. I felt like the world was closing in one me. The day before I was told that I had HIV I had a test so I could become a nurse in the navy. Now I needed to abandon these plans and start combination therapy treatment for HIV.

Initially I dealt with HIV all by myself. It was a one woman journey. I hid in my job, worked out at the gym, and when I wasn't doing anything, the four walls of my room were my refuge. I found comfort in reading novels. I didn't cry or release any emotion.

This took its toll. I developed illnesses and side-effects I'd never heard of before and became depressed. I ended up leaving my job.

Then my health advisor referred me to a support organisation called Living Well.

Six months after finding out that I had HIV, I told my aunt. She's my next of kin. She took it okay, but she was not happy.

But going to Living Well with HIV I met people who have had HIV for 15 or even 20 years. I began to become more comfortable about having HIV, and was working hard and taking care of myself and going to the gym.

My viral load is now undetectable and my CD4 cell count is 208. I've just done a self-management course and it's given me an insight into what I want to do next - I'd like to work with people with chronic illnesses.

Unfortunately my brain tumour came back in November 2005 - part of all the stress of my HIV diagnosis. I really don't know if I am in control. It's been very hard finding out that I have two chronic illnesses in the space of a year - there've been times when I haven't wanted to live past 30, but at other times I want to get involved with people and put back something I've learnt from my own experiences.

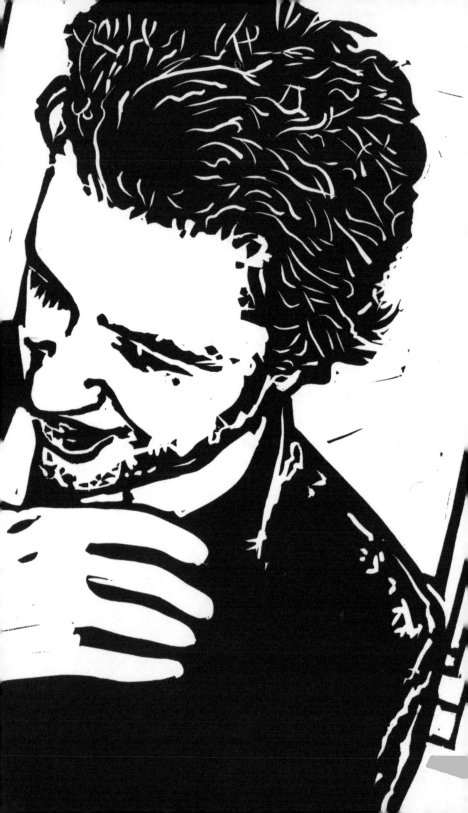

HIV, the basics

In this chapter you'll find information on

The difference between HIV and AIDS.

How HIV is transmitted.

What the HIV test looks for.

The different stages of HIV infection.

How anti-HIV treatment can mean a longer
and healthier life.

There are two testimonies, one from a
woman and one from a man, explaining how
HIV has affected attitudes towards their
life-expectancy.

HIV

HIV stands for human immunodeficiency virus. It was identified in the early 1980s, and belongs to a group of viruses called retroviruses.

HIV prevents the body's immune system from working properly. Normally, the immune system would fight off an infection, but HIV infects key cells in the body's natural defences called CD4 cells, which co-ordinate the body's response to infection. Many CD4 cells are killed by being infected, and others, including some cells that remain uninfected, stop working properly.

AIDS

Over time, the gradual weakening of the immune system leaves the body vulnerable to serious infections and cancers which it would normally be able to fight off. These are called 'opportunistic infections' because they take the opportunity of the body's weakened immunity to take hold.

If you develop certain opportunistic infections, you are diagnosed as having AIDS. AIDS stands for Acquired Immune Deficiency Syndrome. Different people diagnosed as having AIDS may become unwell with different illnesses, depending on the specific opportunistic infections they develop. This is why AIDS is not considered a disease, but a syndrome - a collection of different signs and symptoms, all caused by the same virus, HIV.

HIV transmission

HIV is present in the blood, semen and vaginal fluids of infected people, and can only be passed on to another person if these fluids get into his or her body. Although HIV has been found in the saliva of some people with HIV using very sensitive laboratory equipment, it is in such small quantities that it is not infectious.

The main ways HIV is transmitted are:

- By anal or vaginal sex without a condom. HIV cannot pass through good-quality condoms, and the failure rate of properly used condoms is extremely low.

- Through blood-to-blood contact. This mainly happens through sharing infected drug injecting equipment. In the past, before screening was introduced, some people were infected with blood and blood products during medical treatment. Very rarely, healthcare workers have been infected after accidentally pricking themselves with a needle contaminated with HIV-infected blood.

- From a mother to her baby. This is also called vertical transmission, and can happen during pregnancy, birth or breastfeeding.

Detailed information on HIV transmission can be found in the sections on *Sex and HIV* and *Mother-to-baby transmission of HIV*.

The HIV test

HIV infection is normally detected using an HIV antibody test. This test looks for the antibodies the immune system produces to fight HIV infection. It is very accurate.

The overwhelming majority of people infected with HIV will produce antibodies within 45 days of infection. Some people produce antibodies sooner, and in a very small number of people it can take six months, or even longer, for antibodies to appear after infection.

The HIV antibody test is not an 'AIDS test'. There is no such thing.

Tests can also be used to look for HIV itself (an antigen test) or parts of its genetic material (a PCR - polymerase chain reaction - test), often called a viral load test. Viral load testing is covered in a lot more detail in the section *Key tests to monitor HIV - CD4 and viral load*.

Stages of HIV infection

Becoming HIV antibody positive - seroconversion

Some people have a short illness soon after infection, called a 'seroconversion illness' because it coincides with the period during which the body first produces antibodies to HIV. Common symptoms include a fever lasting more than a few days, aching limbs, a blotchy red rash, headache, diarrhoea and mouth ulcers.

The severity of symptoms can vary considerably between people - they can be so mild as to go unnoticed or so severe that admission to hospital is required. It's now thought that the longer and more severe the symptoms, the greater your chance of developing AIDS within five years, presuming that you do not take anti-HIV drugs.

Doctors are currently trying to see if taking anti-HIV treatment soon after you are infected with HIV is of any long-term benefit. You can find out more and about HIV treatments in the section *Anti-HIV treatment*.

HIV infection without symptoms

Initially, any effects which HIV is having on the immune system don't cause outward signs or symptoms. For this reason, this period is called 'asymptomatic HIV infection' and it can last for months or several years.

But even if you are feeling 100% well, HIV might be damaging your immune system. Doctors use two key laboratory tests to see how active HIV is and what impact it is having on your immune system. These tests are a CD4 cell count, which gives a rough indication of the strength of the immune system, and an HIV viral load test, which shows how active HIV is in the body. Both these tests are discussed in a lot more detail in the section *Key tests to monitor HIV - CD4 and viral load*.

Sometimes you may notice that your glands, or lymph nodes, in various parts of your body become and stay swollen. This is called PGL, or Persistent Generalised Lymphadenopathy. This can happen when you've no other symptoms, and isn't a sign that you are becoming unwell or are at increased risk of doing so in the near future.

HIV infection with symptoms

The longer you live with HIV without treatment, the greater your risk of developing symptoms. These can be caused by infections that take advantage of your weakened immunity, certain cancers and/or the direct effects that HIV can have on the body.

An AIDS diagnosis

If you have certain serious infections or cancers which have been confirmed by tests, then you will be diagnosed as having AIDS. In the US, if your CD4 cell count falls to below 200, the level at which you become vulnerable to serious infections, you are also diagnosed as having AIDS.

More than a definition

A model for describing HIV progression has developed to suggest that there is an inevitable, one-way course in HIV infection. It implies that everybody with HIV will be initially well, then get abnormal CD4 and viral load tests before becoming ill with minor illnesses, and finally go on to develop severe and fatal illness.

This has been the pattern for many people, but others have had very different experiences. For example, some people have had an illness which has led to them being diagnosed with AIDS, and then completely recovered and lived for many years, even decades, in very good health. What's more, many people who have had HIV for many years have never experienced any illness or disease because of HIV.

HIV treatments - the changed reality of living with HIV

The continuous development of new and improved medical treatment both for HIV and the illnesses it can cause has led to major changes in the pattern of HIV disease progression which people in the UK and other rich countries can expect to experience.

First of all, doctors became very skilled at treating some AIDS-defining illnesses. For example, the pneumonia PCP was often fatal in the very early days of the HIV epidemic. Now, doctors are able to control it, and people who have had it go on to live healthy lives for many years afterwards.

What's more, doctors know how to prevent many infections from occurring in the first place. Once your immune system becomes damaged to such an extent that you are vulnerable to certain infections, it is possible to take medicines to prevent these developing. This is called prophylaxis. It's considered in more detail in the section *Symptoms and illnesses*.

However, the biggest improvement of all came in the mid-1990s, when effective treatment that targets HIV itself became available. These antiretroviral treatments have led to very substantial reductions in the numbers of people dying of HIV or becoming ill because of HIV in the UK and similar countries. Use of antiretroviral drugs has been shown to prevent peoples' immune systems from becoming weakened by HIV. What's more, antiretroviral therapy has also been shown to work for many people with advanced HIV disease, including people with AIDS, for many of whom anti-HIV drugs have brought about a remarkable recovery in health.

Treatments for HIV are considered in a lot more detail in the chapter *Anti-HIV treatment.*

Prognosis

The prognosis for people with HIV has changed dramatically since the first cases of AIDS were diagnosed in the early 1980s. In those early days, it was thought that most people would die within a few months of first being diagnosed with the condition. This changed, partly because it was recognised that HIV was the cause of AIDS and that it took many years to gradually destroy the immune system, and partly because doctors gradually learnt more about recognising and treating infections and cancers commonly seen in people with HIV. By the mid-1990s (before the introduction of effective anti-HIV treatment), it was thought that in rich countries such as the UK it would take between eight and fifteen years (on average) after infection with the virus for HIV to cause life-threatening illness or death.

Many HIV doctors now believe that provided a person with HIV receives effective anti-HIV treatment before their immune system has been severely damaged by the virus, and if they take their drugs properly and can tolerate them, they could live a more or less normal life span.

The use of Highly Active Antiretroviral Therapy (HAART; combinations of drugs which slow down the rate at which HIV is able to reproduce) from the mid-1990s onwards has led to dramatic improvements in the prognosis for people with HIV. For instance, AIDS deaths in the UK have fallen from a peak of over 1,500 in 1994 to approximately 400 a year at present. The AIDS deaths which still occur in this country often involve people who are diagnosed with HIV late in the disease process, when their immune system is already severely damaged.

Research into the prognosis of people starting HIV treatment indicates that the risk of becoming very ill or dying because of HIV within the next three years is linked to five key factors: having a CD4 count below 200 or a viral load above 100,000 at the time of starting treatment; being aged over 50; being an injecting drug user; or having had a prior AIDS-defining illness.

In the UK it is recommended that anti-HIV treatment is started before your CD4 count falls below 200, which is an indication that HIV has damaged your immune system to such an extent that you are vulnerable to serious illness. It is also strongly recommended that you start anti-HIV drugs if you become ill because of HIV. Starting treatment in these circumstances has been shown to improve prognosis compared to delaying treatment until later.

You can find out more about when to start HIV treatments in the section *Anti-HIV treatment*.

Some non-AIDS-related illnesses occur more frequently in people with HIV, despite the effectiveness of HIV treatment. These include liver disease caused by hepatitis viruses B or C; certain cancers, such as lung cancer, testicular cancer, cervical cancer and anal cancer; and mental illnesses such as depression. In addition, HIV treatments themselves can cause long-term side-effects which can seriously affect health or quality of life.

There's more information on hepatitis B and C in the section on *Symptoms and illnesses*, and depression is considered in a lot more detail in the section on *Mental health*. The section *Side-effects* provides a lot more information about these.

Obviously, there are many other causes of ill health apart from HIV, and so more general health advice (such as stopping smoking, taking regular exercise, eating a balanced diet) is also relevant to people with HIV. To find out more about these issues, read the section *Daily health issues*.

Further reading
- NAM factsheets, *Infectiousness, HIV's lifecycle* and *Prognosis*.
- 'Introduction to HIV and AIDS' in NAM's *HIV and AIDS Treatment Directory*.
- *Protecting you - a basic guide to your immune system*, booklet produced by the Terrence Higgins Trust.
- *Tell me about HIV,* booklet produced by the UK Coalition of People Living With HIV and AIDS.

The bus of doom

by Caroline Guinness

I've recently read the His Dark Materials trilogy by Philip Pullman (which, if you haven't already read, I highly recommend). In this theological novel disguised as a children's book, a group of kids are pursued through parallel universes.

I was struck by the concept, as we have recently moved from London to rural Wiltshire, and the contrast between the two is obvious. I grew up on a farm in Cape Town and had wanted to get out of London for many years, as I feel so much more at home in the country.

But quite aside from my daughter being at school in London and having all her friends there, I was too nervous to stray far from my HIV clinic.

Once I did fall seriously ill, while staying with friends near here. Rather than face the local A&E, I got into my car and drove 200 miles to the Royal Free in north London. I promptly passed out in the waiting room and on coming to was asked how I got there. I said that I had driven from Dorset. They gasped. "But Caroline, you have a temperature of 104 and E-coli septicaemia!" "Yes," I answered, "That's why I drove here."

But now I've had six years of successful anti-HIV treatment, married a fabulous man, and my daughter is at university in America. So I thought it was time to take the plunge and go back to my country roots. Through a friend, we found a gorgeous 400-year-old thatched house on a country estate near Salisbury, and four weeks ago we moved in. I promptly forgot about HIV, and telling the locals about it seems not so much impossible as irrelevant. I will drive up every three months for the usual check-up at my clinic and catch up with friends at the same time, but almost instantly I felt the stress fall away. Our two dogs and cat think they have landed up in paradise. We do not need to drive to the nearest park for a walk - it is right outside our front door.

Everything was perfect until my daughter returned for a break, and we decided to drive to London so she could catch up with friends. Setting off on a sunny day, we got to a crossroads just outside the nearest village, where there is a completely blind corner. I edged the car out so I could look to my left and was promptly hit by a bus driving at around 60 miles an hour.

It all happened in a second. I blacked out for a few minutes and came round to find the airbags in our faces and smoke pouring out of the car. How we stepped out alive I don't know. The car was a complete write-off and the bus missed my daughter by inches.

Other than a few bruises, we seemed to be physically OK, but the shock was indescribable. In the midst of it all, however, I found myself laughing. In all the years of having HIV, the one thing that drove me completely mad was the old phrase: "Yes, but everyone dies one day. You never know, you could be hit by a bus!"

I would try to explain that being diagnosed with a terminal illness was very different, and anyway, how many people did they know who had ever actually been hit by a bus?

Well, I have now. Here I am, 16 years after diagnosis, eleven years past the sell-by date I was originally given, still alive, still HIV-positive, but no longer in a position to feel anger at one particular unthinking remark. Next time someone mentions being hit by that bus I'll say, "Well, I already have, actually."

I am now getting country sympathy about the appalling driving of the local bus drivers, speed limits on country roads and how this corner has been a notorious black spot for years. Also the odd condescending remark, such as, " Oh well, now you know that driving is different here in the country. You'll have to adjust." Parallel universes, indeed. Takes the mind off HIV, anyway.

This first appeared in issue 80/81 of Positive Nation, July/August 2002. Many thanks to both Caroline and Positive Nation for giving permission to reprint it here.

20 years and counting

I became infected in 1984 and this month celebrated the fact that not only was it my 51st birthday, but also I had survived twenty years with HIV. On the weekend of my 31st birthday I received an unwanted gift, which unfortunately could not be taken back and exchanged for vouchers. I have thus spent the major portion of my adult life with the virus underlying almost every decision and action. Prognosis for me in early 1985 was that "another six months" was unlikely and that I should ensure that "my affairs were in order".

I have survived, I believe, through a combination of factors; good luck probably being the most relevant. I have been enormously lucky for the unconditional acceptance and love that I have received from my family and friends and the depth and quality of medical support that I have been privileged to obtain. I've worked hard at it as well; not prepared to give up in what is simply an instinctive fight for survival.

Nobody needs telling that life ain't easy. Fear, depression and loneliness were almost constant companions, but there were lots of good times too. I got into a very intimate and enduring relationship with alcohol, from which I have eventually managed to extract myself. Life and some degree of sanity somehow survived that affair, but it was a very close call at times.

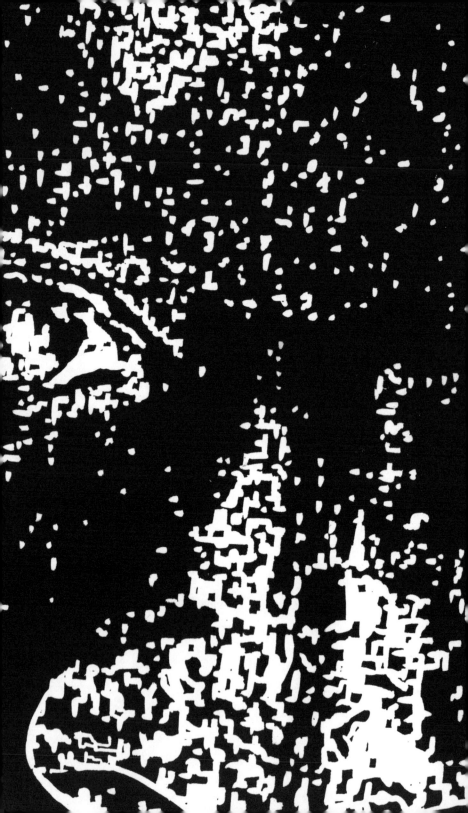

Telling people you are HIV-positive

In this chapter you'll find information on

Issues you may want to consider before you
tell people you are HIV-positive.

Telling partners, family, friends, colleagues
and healthcare staff that you have HIV.

There are two testimonies, one by a woman
and the other by a man, on their
experiences of telling their partner and
friends that they had HIV.

Don't rush

Telling people that you have HIV can seem like a daunting or even frightening task. It's important to think about who you are going to tell, and your motivation for telling them. There are lots of reasons why you might want to tell people that you have HIV, not least the valuable support which your partner (if you have one), family and friends might be able to provide. But don't rush into telling people - although you can tell people you have HIV later, you cannot un-tell somebody.

On first learning that you have HIV, or later, when you perhaps receive bad test results, you may feel a desire to unburden yourself and tell somebody. However, you may regret this later. Although you might want people to know what you are going through at times like this so you can receive their support, there are other times when you might find this intrusive - you may not want to be asked constant questions about your health, how you are feeling or how you are coping. It might even feel that you are finding yourself supporting and reassuring the people who you told about your HIV.

We all react to difficult and stressful situations in different ways. Similarly, there's no rule of thumb about what sort of support you should ask from those close to you. Think about what's best for you. The most important thing is that you feel you have control over who you tell about your HIV.

Practicalities

If you decide to tell somebody that you have HIV, think carefully about what you are going to tell them, and how, where and when you are going to do this. Also think about how they are going to react and prepare to answer questions that you think they might ask you.

Be clear about who they can and cannot share information about your HIV status with. You don't want to lose control over who knows that you have HIV.

Telling somebody that you have HIV might tap into their prejudices about sexuality, illness, disability, race or HIV itself. Think about how you will react if this happens.

It can be very difficult if the person you tell is very upset or doesn't understand. You might feel like the one offering support. In addition, it's possible that a person may feel under pressure to offer you support and may not be able to, or know how to.

Telling your partner

If you have spent time discussing having an HIV test with your partner, then you may have a good idea of what their reaction might be. If you didn't discuss this, then think about the practicalities of telling your partner and what their reaction might be. It could be that your HIV status could have health implications for your partner. Your partner might be a wonderful source of support and love. But on the other hand, telling your partner you have HIV could also put stress on your relationship.

Telling sexual partners

See the section on disclosing your HIV status to sexual partners in the chapter *HIV and the law*.

Telling ex-partners

It can be very difficult telling ex-partners and past sexual contacts that you have HIV. Whether or not you can, or even need to, tell them can depend on a

> The first time I cried was when I told my ex-boyfriend. I knew it would break his heart. He just looked at me and said, "I'm sorry." We hugged and he has stayed my best friend ever since.
>
> positive voice

number of factors, such as what your relationship was like with them, the kind of sex you had, whether you think they would want to know and whether you want them to know.

Staff at your HIV clinic can contact your ex-partners and sexual contacts without giving any of your details away.

Family
You may immediately want to tell your family that you have HIV. However, many people find this very difficult. Breaking the news to your family can be distressing for both you and them. There's no right or wrong time to tell your parents, brothers or sisters that you have HIV. Some people tell them immediately, others after years, and some people never tell their family. You know best what and/or when they would like to know, and how and when to tell them.

Friends
It is good to have somebody close to you to confide in when you are upset, confused, angry, or need to talk things through. You may well have a friend who you instinctively know you can trust to tell that you have HIV and to look for support. But you should still take time to think things through. Think about why you want to tell a friend or friends. Consider the likely impact on your friendship of telling them you have HIV. Think about how they may react when you tell them, and about what their reaction would be if they found out from another source after you didn't tell them.

Remember, friends might talk amongst themselves or to other people about your health. It's important to make it clear to them if you want them to keep information about your HIV to themselves.

Work
In most cases, there should be no reason why your employer would need to know that you have HIV. Even if you need to have a lot off time off sick, there is no need for your employer to know that HIV is the cause.

Some employers offer very good support to people with HIV, and the UK Disability Discrimination Act makes it illegal for an HIV-positive person to be discriminated against at work because of their health status, from the moment of their diagnosis.

Healthcare professionals

GPs

Everybody who is HIV-positive should be registered with a GP. In order for your GP to provide the most appropriate care, it is important that they know if you have any serious medical conditions, including HIV, or are taking medicines that a hospital specialist has prescribed to you, such as anti-HIV medication.

GPs are not allowed to refuse to register you because you are HIV-positive, or discriminate against you in any way because you are HIV-positive or because of your sexuality, sex or lifestyle.

A lot of people are concerned that informing their GP that they have HIV could have implications if they apply for a mortgage or life assurance. Your GP records are confidential, but it is true that if you apply for life cover the company will almost certainly ask about your medical history and ask to have access to your GP records. You should be aware, however, that if you fail to tell a life insurance company that you are HIV-positive when you apply for a home loan it could have very serious consequences later.

Your HIV clinic may have a list of recommended GPs in your area.

Dentists

When you register with a dentist, you may be asked to fill out a form describing your medical history. This may ask you if you are HIV-positive and have certain other illnesses such as hepatitis B or C. Alternatively, a dentist may ask you if you're HIV-positive.

According to the professional body for UK dentists, a dentist should not discriminate against you because you disclose your HIV status. Sadly, this has not always been the case. Dentists have sometimes claimed that they have refused treatment in order to protect themselves and their other patients from HIV. This is not acceptable. Standard sterilisation and infection control procedures are sufficient to ensure that no patient poses a risk to dental staff or other patients.

Telling your dentist you have HIV can have benefits. They can check for certain gum problems that can occur more often in people with HIV. Also, it is wise to tell your dentist if you are taking any medication prescribed to treat HIV or any other infections, as dentists may need to use drugs that could interact with them.

If you are worried about telling a dentist, then ask your HIV clinic to recommend one. They may even have a specialist HIV dentist. Your dental records are confidential.

Pharmacists

A pharmacist may ask you what medicines you are taking when they dispense a prescription or when you buy over-the-counter medication. Some over-the-counter medicines (medicines available without a doctor's prescription), for example hay fever tablets, can interact dangerously with certain anti-HIV drugs. It can be especially hard to maintain your

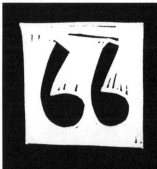

When I first knew my husband was HIV-positive, I wasn't sure who to turn to and I told some parents at my children's school. The next thing I knew, the head teacher had received an anonymous phone call saying that I was HIV-positive and that I shouldn't be allowed to help out at school. Fortunately, the head was very supportive, but I worried for months about other parents, other children in the playground and maybe even our children finding out.

positive voice

confidentiality at a high street pharmacy counter, so if you do need over-the-counter medicines on a regular basis, it might be wise to discuss this with your HIV doctor or specialist HIV pharmacist.

Complementary health practitioners

Many people with HIV use complementary therapists, such as acupuncturists. If you do, you may wish to disclose your health status to them. It should not make a difference to the kind of therapy they offer you.

However, complementary practitioners are not as well regulated as medical professionals. You may wish to check confidentiality policies before disclosing any health details.

If you are advised to take any complementary or alternative therapy, check with your doctor or HIV pharmacist that it is safe. Some alternative medicines, such as the herbal anti-depressant St John's wort, can stop some anti-HIV drugs working properly. Even if you tell a complementary practitioner that you are taking anti-HIV drugs, it is not certain that they will know of any possible dangerous interactions.

Children

Children can be very perceptive and might be worrying if their parent or guardian is ill. They need clear and appropriate information to help them understand the situation.

You may find that even very young children will want to know why their parent has to go to the doctor a lot or is constantly unwell. It could be useful to talk about "goodies" or "baddies" in the blood, or bugs, which may enable you to talk about illness without actually mentioning HIV. In this way, you can begin to foster an understanding of health and illness which you can build upon, adding more details as the child gets older.

Further reading

- NAM factsheet, *Disclosing your HIV status to healthcare workers.*
- *Should I Tell,* Booklet produced by Terrence Higgins Trust.

Grateful? I don't think so
by Susan

"You must be so grateful that your partner agreed to stay with you despite the fact that you have, you know, AIDS," said a particularly vacuous journalist to me, during an interview for a women's magazine. "Actually, no," I replied, "He's grateful that I stay with him, because I'm so great in bed." Strangely, she chose to ignore my comment and continued to portray me as a vapid pathetic creature, ashamed of my status and gushing with gratitude that someone would deign to go out with diseased old me. No mention of the fact that I have a remarkable capacity to suppress my gag reflex.

It saddens me when I read about people living with HIV who feel that they have to hang up their shagging shoes and turn to a life of laborious abstinence. Should an HIV-positive diagnosis correlate with an abandoned libido? Well, I must confess that I did have a temporary loss of libido when I was first diagnosed. Being told that I only had four years to live didn't make me feel particularly horny. Perhaps feeling that sex was the cause of my being HIV-positive, coupled with my Catholic conscience issues, put me off the dirty deed for a while.

At the time, I was in a relationship with a particularly vile American. He suggested that no one would want to be with me now, as I was HIV-positive. My self-esteem was so suppressed that I actually believed him. After we split up, I felt that my life would comprise of eating microwave meals for one and masturbation (surprisingly pleasurable if undertaken simultaneously). It took a year of making my eyesight considerably worse (only kidding), before I abandoned that notion.

I met my current partner at a conference and was immediately blinded with lust. I initially believed that our relationship would simply be a short-term sex thing, so didn't feel that it was necessary to disclose my status - we always had protected sex. A month later, I found myself in the heinous position of falling in love. I vacillated with the idea of dumping him, rather than face being rejected when I told him about my positive status. Finally I chose to tell him, classily, in a McDonald's car park (the rationale being that, if he rejected me, I'd have the compensation of a Big Mac Meal).

I began in a somewhat cowardly way, by saying "I have something to tell you about me, that's quite bad", and proceeded to let him guess. His first guess, rather alarmingly, was that I used to be a man - but he finally got there. Instead of rushing off to scrub himself in bleach, he professed his love, and five years later we're still together.

I do hope we'll stay together long-term, but if we don't, I don't think I'll be booking myself into the nearest nunnery quite yet. My self-esteem has rebounded to its previous monstrous proportions - to the extent that I believe most men would be lucky to have me, regardless of my HIV-positive status. Pass me a banana and I'll show you one of the reasons why.

Telling people
by Alan

The lunch time after finding out I had HIV, I called a colleague who was also a close friend. I had planned just to make sure I could see her in the evening when I got back to town. But she could hear something terrible in my voice and asked whether something was wrong. I admitted there was, but still didn't want to tell her the shocking news on the phone. It had to be carefully done and I had hardly absorbed the reality. But it blurted out, and this first person I had chosen to tell I knew was strong in a crisis. Nevertheless, I found myself reassuring her that I was coping while seeking assurance that we would meet that night and talk it through.

A few weeks after finding out that I had HIV I told my aunt, the family member to whom I felt the closest.

Why tell anyone? Because I thought I was going to die young (this was back in 1990, before effective anti-HIV treatment was available). I thought it was going to be a terrible death, covered in sores, wasting away with a deadly disease which was thought then to be so easily transmitted. How could I not tell the people who really loved me? However upsetting it was going to be, for us both, how much worse for them to have to be told when it becomes obvious that things were dire. If your meaningful relationships are based on truth, how then can you allow in a mammoth lie? I imagined them reckoning what the real value of our love was if I had protected them from the truth until the last possible moment, however well meaning my intentions. Why had I not given them the opportunity to love me and care for me through my ordeal? Love is not just for the good times.

Also, quite selfishly, I needed to tell some people. I needed their care. I needed them to know so that they could prepare for helping me through the worst. I needed people I could trust to talk through all the issues and implications. I wasn't strong enough to do this on my own

After careful thought, my aunt's brilliant response was to clear my quite substantial debts as something to reduce stress. This allowed me to give up being a lawyer and find less stressful work. I wasn't going to give up on life until I had to, but I was going to make it less strenuous. Reducing stress was a treatment without risk.

A few months later, for the same twin reasons of need for honesty and support, I decided to tell my parents. They were retired, less worldly than my aunt, and there was the fear of what the shock would do to them. But they would have wanted to know and have the opportunity to do what they could to help. I travelled down to see them for a weekend with that friend I'd first told. At least I had all the then information at my finger tips and I could explain it to them as calmly as possible, but I also needed that friend with me. She was able to spend her own time talking with my folks. For them to hear the information again calmly from a third person would help them. It would help me. Having to take some control of immediate emotions a little in front of a relatively unknown person would help the stiff upper lip. There were still lots of tears of course. It's a big thing to hear that your only child has probably only very few years to live; but they coped. Their main concern was how they could help.

The next person I told was my then lover. Again, you cannot have a successful relationship built upon a lie, but I also wanted him to be able to make the choices about a future together with full knowledge of the issues. As it happened, he left me after only a few months but not because of the HIV; he hadn't sorted out his own sexuality.

I have not told many people, and I have never had a bad reaction. Only very close friends and family know. I think they are the only people who should, or need to know. One exception was an ex-colleague and neighbour who was going through a very stressful time because of an unwanted divorce. She was desperately unhappy and grieving her loss. Perversely perhaps, I chose to tell her of my burden, which at the time still meant an early death, so as to try to put her ordeal into some context. It worked. I've never told an employer and thus have had to lie on some forms. There is still so much ignorance out there about the virus. Similarly I've avoided any further health or life insurance so as to avoid making a false declaration.

Two weeks after we started going out, I told my current partner. I took him for a walk in the park and sitting on a bench in the sunshine told him the truth. He cried, not just for me but also for him; because he said he wished we had met earlier so that we could have had longer together. Lucky me, he is still my partner after over twelve years and our Civil Partnership is at the end of this month. We've lived a full life.

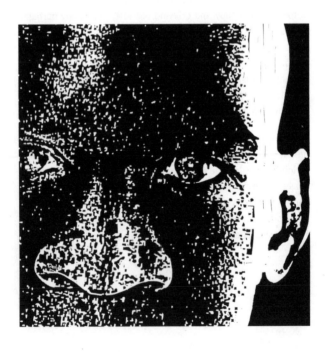

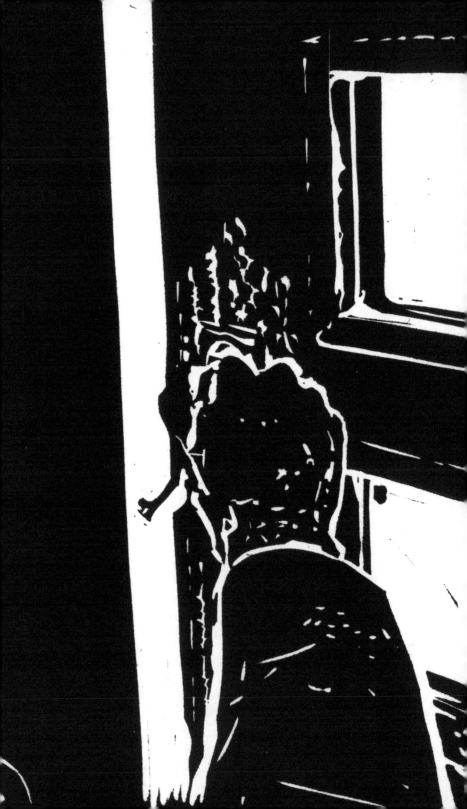

Getting HIV treatment and care

In this chapter you'll find information on

HIV clinics, how to find one, and what you can expect from them.

Your relationship with your doctor.

GPs and dentists.

NHS care and people who are not from the UK.

There is a testimony from an HIV-positive asylum seeker.

In the UK, nearly all HIV treatment and care is provided by specialist hospital clinics. Because HIV has mainly (but not exclusively) been spread through sex in this country, HIV healthcare services in the UK developed through, and are often provided by, genitourinary medicine (GUM) and sexual health clinics. In some parts of the UK, infectious disease or immunology departments developed into specialist HIV clinics. HIV clinics may also be provided through haematology units for people with haemophilia, drug dependency units for injecting drug users, and specialist children's hospitals.

Many HIV treatment centres are in London. This is because the majority of people with HIV live in London. However, there are hospitals offering HIV treatment and care in all the major cities in the UK.

HIV clinics

HIV care is provided through outpatient clinics. This means that you do not receive your treatment whilst staying in hospital, but visit a specialist doctor at regular intervals who will monitor your health, prescribe treatments and, if you need to, refer you to see other specialists.

Many HIV clinics are attached to a GUM clinic, and there's a good chance that you will be receiving your HIV care from the HIV clinic associated with the GUM clinic where you were diagnosed with HIV.

Unlike any other specialism within the NHS, GUM and HIV clinics operate an open access policy. You don't need your family doctor to refer you. All you have to do is phone up and make an appointment. You can choose which HIV treatment centre you receive your care from. You do not have to attend the clinic at the hospital you were diagnosed at. If you wish, you can use the HIV treatment centre in a different city. If you decide to change clinics, it's very important to ensure that your medical notes are forwarded from your old clinic to your new one.

If you are entitled to free NHS care, then all the treatment you receive from your HIV clinic will be free. Even if you normally have to pay for prescriptions, nearly all medicines prescribed by a specialist HIV doctor will be free.

It's likely that, as well as regular appointments with a doctor who specialises in the treatment of HIV, your clinic will have other specialist services available to you. There will almost certainly be a specialist HIV pharmacist. There's also a good chance that there are nurse-led clinics looking after sexual health, or supporting adherence to drug regimens. The very large HIV clinics may also have specialist HIV mental health teams, and access to dentists.

An emergency walk-in doctor service is provided by some clinics during normal working hours. This is intended for problems requiring urgent medical attention.

Opening times vary between clinics. You can expect the very large clinics to be open and to offer appointments with doctors and other health professionals every working day. By contrast, smaller clinics might only be open a few mornings or afternoons a week.

All clinics will have arrangements for providing emergency care. The large HIV clinics will have an HIV doctor who is on call 24 hours a day for an emergency, while at smaller hospitals emergency cover might be provided by a general medicine doctor.

The factors influencing choice of clinic differ from person to person. Some might prefer to attend a clinic that is large, with a reputation for expertise. Others opt to attend smaller clinics that are more accessible and convenient.

Whichever clinic you attend, it's very important that you receive appropriate treatment and care that you are comfortable with. If you are not satisfied with the level of service you are receiving, then complain to the clinic management. Set out clearly what you are unhappy about. An advocacy organisation such as the UK Coalition of People Living with HIV and AIDS might be able to help. Try not to get angry, and don't get abusive. The chances are that your complaint will be settled satisfactorily. If your complaint isn't settled to your satisfaction, then remember you can change to a different clinic.

Your HIV clinic will also have facilities to treat inpatients (treatment whilst staying in hospital). Large clinics are likely to have a dedicated HIV ward with doctors and nurses who only treat HIV-positive patients. If you attend a smaller clinic, then inpatient care is likely to be provided on a general medical or infectious diseases ward.

Staff on specialist inpatient wards may well have more insight into the medical and psychological issues faced by people with HIV, and will have more skill at recognising and treating both the common and uncommon illnesses and complications seen in people with HIV. Other staff at hospitals with a large HIV clinic, such as pharmacists, dieticians, radiologists and physiotherapists will also have extensive experience of treating HIV-positive patients.

It's worth bearing in mind that the large HIV clinics, which have lots of patients and more expertise, have better survival and outcome rates for their patients. To put it simply: if you go to a large clinic with experienced staff, you improve your chances of living a longer, healthier life.

If you are admitted to hospital for a reason unconnected to HIV, it's very important to let the doctors and nurses looking after you know that you are HIV-positive, to ensure that you receive the right treatment.

You and your doctor

The relationship you forge with your specialist HIV doctor is one of the most important you will have after your diagnosis.

Certain doctors may attract certain kinds of patients: some doctors will advocate aggressive therapy, whilst others will be more receptive should you wish to hold off treatment or use a range of complementary approaches in addition to conventional HIV care.

It's important that you find the right kind of doctor for you. Friends who are HIV-positive may be able to recommend a suitable doctor, but building up a relationship will take time. You may not develop a rapport with the first doctor you meet. Establishing a trusting relationship with your doctor is essential if you are to feel empowered and in control of your use of treatments.

Your doctor should have good interpersonal skills. The level of knowledge of your clinician is clearly important too. An effective doctor should take the trouble to explain things to you, be sensitive to personal issues raised by you, be a good listener and be able to provide you with a range of opinions.

All patients need their doctors to be open, frank and communicative - as well as honest when he or she does not know the answer to your questions.

You will need to be involved in your own care. Exactly what this means depends upon the type of person you are. Some people will want to take a more active role in their healthcare. They may have clear ideas about what kind of treatments they do or do not want to use. Others will be more inclined to look to their doctor for guidance.

Being prepared for your consultations is a joint responsibility. Keep asking questions until you understand. If you are likely to forget what your doctor tells you during the consultation, make notes. If you are likely to forget which questions you would like to ask, then write a letter to your doctor containing the questions you want to ask, and send it in advance of your appointment. It's also worth remembering that if you attend your clinic without an appointment, your regular doctor may not be available.

During the course of your relationship with your doctor, there will probably occasionally be issues upon which you do not agree. It's important that you learn how to manage these situations. If you become unhappy over a disagreement with your doctor, you may choose to invite a patient advocate to help you communicate your feelings.

It is important to be honest with your doctor about any risks you may be taking, or sexual practices, alcohol or drug use that may affect your long-term health. Knowing the facts helps your doctor to consider appropriate care and treatment for you. If, however, you feel unable to confide in your doctor about certain issues, there may be other staff in the department who you could talk to more easily.

Maintaining contact with the same doctor can be extremely difficult, as they are usually very busy, and staff change from time to time. Remember though, their time is no more valuable than your own. If getting access to your doctor is difficult, discuss ways of improving the situation. Would a short phone call or email enquiry be acceptable? You will need to be organised to get the most from your doctor's time. Learning about the roles of other staff at your treatment centre will also help you avoid using your doctor's time when another member of staff would be able to help, and can provide you with additional sources of support. For some non-HIV-related medical problems, it might be more appropriate to see a GP.

GPs

Even though you receive your HIV care from a specialist HIV clinic, it is still important to have a GP. Firstly, many GPs offer services which are not available at your HIV clinic, but which you may need from time to time, such as health visiting for women who have recently had a baby; district nurses, if you need nursing support at home; mental health nursing; physiotherapy and chiropody.

GPs are able to provide prescriptions for non-HIV medicines which your clinic may be unable to supply for more than a couple of weeks. Also, GPs are the only doctors who can make home visits if you are too ill to attend your HIV clinic or your GP's surgery. If you are unwell outside normal working hours, or at the weekend or bank holidays, all GPs have an emergency service through which a nurse or doctor will offer advice and, if necessary, visit you at home. If the problem is very serious and requires

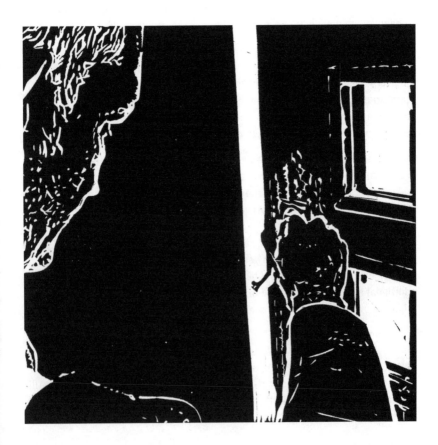

hospital care, they can arrange for your admission into hospital and will normally be willing to speak to the on-call HIV doctor at your clinic to arrange specialist HIV care if appropriate.

To get access to a GP you must be registered as their patient. You can only be registered with one GP and you must live within the area the GP practices in. When you register you will be asked to give your name and address, your NHS number and details of your last GP. Don't worry if you can't find your NHS number, you can still register without it. A few weeks after you register with a GP you will receive a card confirming your registration, which will have your NHS number on it.

Most HIV clinics keep a list of GPs, and may be able to recommend a GP with experience of caring for people with HIV. However, GPs often find that they cannot accept any more patients, as they already have on their register the maximum number of people to whom they can offer services. You can also contact NHS Direct on 0845 4647 for details of all GP practices in your area. If you still have problems finding a GP who is able to register you, then contact your local Patient Advice and Liaison Service. GPs cannot refuse to register you because you have HIV or any other medical condition, or because of your race, colour or sexuality. It's also worth remembering that many GPs, particularly those with practices outside cities and big towns, may have a very limited knowledge of HIV and will have seen very few HIV-positive patients.

If you need a GP when you are away from home, then you can register as a 'temporary resident' if you will be within their practice area for 14 days or less.

If you are entitled to free NHS treatment, then all NHS services provided by your GP will be free. GPs are not obliged to provide free NHS treatment to people who are visiting the UK from abroad or who do not have the legal right to stay in the UK. GPs also provide some other services for a fee, such as signing passport applications.

Most GPs have an appointment system, and sometimes these become booked up for weeks in advance. Emergency appointments will usually be available for people who need to be seen quickly. These are normally available the same day, but on a 'first come, first served' basis.

If you don't disclose your HIV status to your GP, you must be aware that this may prevent you from receiving the best care. For example, if you are taking HIV drugs, it's important to consider potentially harmful interactions with other medications. Your GP medical records are confidential, and nobody can see them without your consent. If you are concerned about disclosing your status, explore whether staff at your HIV treatment centre, or an advocate, could help you assess your GP's practice around disclosure beforehand.

Dentists

There have been cases where people with HIV have been refused treatment by a dentist. Dentists in the UK have been told by their governing body that they cannot refuse to treat somebody just because they are HIV-positive. General hygiene precautions are enough to prevent the transmission of HIV during dental treatment.

As with all healthcare workers, it's a good idea to let them know if you have any serious medical conditions or are taking any medication. This will help them ensure that you receive the most appropriate treatment. It is wrong for dentists or any other health professional to discriminate against you because of your health status, race, or sexuality.

Not all dentists offer NHS care, and in some parts of the UK there are long waiting lists to register with NHS dentists.

Your HIV clinic might be able to help you find an NHS dentist, or a dentist that is particularly skilled or interested in treating people with HIV. Some of the large HIV clinics even have their own dental clinics.

Regular visits to the dentist are recommended for people with HIV. Not only will this ensure that your general dental health is being looked after, but it will also allow dentists to look for gum and mouth disorders, such as oral thrush and badly bleeding gums, which can occur more frequently in people with HIV.

NHS care and non-UK nationals

There is no general right to come to the United Kingdom in order to obtain free treatment from the UK's National Health Service (NHS). Nationals of the member states of the European Economic Area (EEA), or their family members, and refugees and stateless persons living within the EEA, have the right to NHS treatment without charge where the need arises during their stay. EEA nationals who wish to enter the UK for treatment (or who are referred to the UK for treatment) should obtain prior authorisation from their national social security institution, which in principle bears the cost, and obtain a European Health Insurance Card before travelling. The EEA member states are: Austria, Belgium, Denmark, Finland, France, Germany, Greece, Iceland, Ireland, Italy, Liechtenstein, Luxembourg, Netherlands, Norway, Portugal, Spain, and Sweden.

Most NHS treatment is not automatically free of charge to other people from abroad. Access to the NHS depends on a combination of one or more of: immigration status; length of residence; nature of the treatment required; and whether the need for it arose during the visit.

However, certain NHS treatment is free to everyone. This includes testing and counselling for HIV or sexually transmitted infections at a genitourinary clinic (but not any subsequent treatment for HIV), family planning services, treatment for mental disorders, hospital accident and emergency treatment

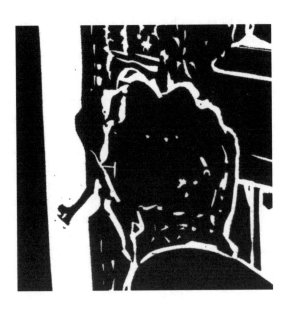

(but not in-patient care) and treatment for notifiable diseases and other conditions to which public health laws apply (not including HIV and AIDS).

In addition, certain categories of people are exempt from any NHS charges. The main categories are: anyone in employment in the UK; anyone taking up permanent residence in the UK; anyone who has resided in the UK for twelve months; refugees and asylum seekers; prisoners and immigration detainees; full-time students; those whose home countries have a reciprocal health agreement with the UK.

Asylum seekers have a right to free HIV treatment for as long as their claim is being considered and this period includes any process of appeals. Furthermore, if an HIV-positive asylum seeker is being seen for HIV treatment and care by the NHS then this treatment can continue free of charge even after an asylum claim is finally denied. But the regulations state that someone whose asylum claim has already failed, or is for other reasons without legal residency status, cannot start accessing free HIV treatment on the NHS.

There is considerable inconsistency in the application of these regulations across the country and much confusion both amongst NHS staff and the public on who has a right to free treatment. There have been several documented examples of people wrongly being denied free treatment and anyone living with HIV who is having difficulty in obtaining free HIV treatment should seek advice and support from local or national HIV support organisations. It should also be noted that the charging regulations described above only apply in England.

There is also confusion on the entitlement to free NHS primary care (for example, in GP practices). Asylum seekers are entitled to register with a GP and access free primary care services like anyone else, as long as they live in the practice area and the practice list is open for new registrations. A practice cannot legally refuse to register a patient who happens to be an asylum seeker if their list is open to other patients. The situation for failed asylum seekers and others without legal residency status is less clear. Whilst they have a right to free emergency or immediately necessary treatment from a GP, it seems to be at the GP's discretion whether or not they are allowed to register with the practice for other primary care services. Again, those people living with HIV who are having problems accessing primary care should seek help from HIV or refugee support organisations.

Other categories of people are exempt from charges for treatment, if the need for it arose during a visit to the UK. This provision is intended to exclude travel to the UK specifically for treatment on the NHS of a pre-existing condition.

Immigration is a complex and specialist topic, and the laws can change frequently. It is essential that anyone seeking information on this subject go to appropriate advice agencies. The following organisations can provide guidance:

- Joint Council for the Welfare of Immigrants
  115 Old St, London EC1V 9JR
  020 251 8706 (advice line).

- Refugee Legal Centre
  153-157 Commercial Road, London, E1 2DA
  020 7780 3220 (advice line)
  Open for individual advice on Mon, Tue, Wed
  and Fri 9.30am - 1.00pm and 2pm - 4pm.

- Immigration Law Practitioners Association
  Lindsey House, 40-42 Charterhouse Street, London EC1M 6JN
  020 7251 8383.

- Immigration and Nationality Directorate
  www. ind.homeoffice.gov.uk.

- Citizens Advice Bureau
  www.citizensadvice.org.uk.

Further reading

- 'The law and HIV,' in NAM's *HIV and AIDS Reference Manual.*
- NAM factsheets: *GPs and primary care, HIV clinic services, NHS and non-UK nationals,* and *You and your doctor.*

Anciciaria's story

I want my experiences to give hope to other people - things do not have to end when you find out that you have HIV.

In 2000 I arrived in the UK from Zimbabwe and in 2001 I started a new relationship with a man from a country where many people have HIV. To help protect ourselves against HIV and sexually transmitted infections we both went for tests. His test for HIV was negative. Mine was positive.

My initial reaction was fear. I thought that having HIV would mean that I would die in two or three years. My brother in Zimbabwe was very supportive and he told me that drugs were available that could help people with HIV live for longer.

Support also came closer to home. My HIV consultant and the nurses at my HIV clinic were very helpful and understanding and they put me in touch with support groups for Africans with HIV.

One of my big concerns was that I thought having HIV meant that I would die without ever having a child. You know, I was 34 when I found out I had HIV, so the biological clock was already ticking. And there is a real expectation in my culture that a woman should have a baby.

At a support group I attended, a speaker from Positively Women explained that it is possible for a woman with HIV to have an HIV-negative baby. I met an HIV-positive man in 2002 and became pregnant.

But six weeks later I was dispersed from London to Manchester. I was very concerned because I'd had a miscarriage shortly before and feared that the stress of dispersal would cause me to miscarry again.

Even though I was HIV-positive and pregnant, I had to find an HIV clinic by myself - I did so using the Yellow Pages.

I'm glad to say that in 2003 I had a very healthy HIV-negative baby. My own health was good and my viral load was low so I only needed to take AZT during the last few months of pregnancy. I was even able to have a vaginal delivery, not a caesarean. My baby took a few doses of AZT after she was born. She is beautiful and very healthy.

My own health is very good - my CD4 cell count did dip when I was pregnant but it is now 580 and my viral load is only 68. My consultant said it would be many years before I need to start HIV treatment.

My immigration status has been a big worry. In 2003 my asylum application was refused - at a time when I was pregnant - and I really did fear that I would be deported. But because I'm from Zimbabwe I was advised to make another application which is still ongoing.

I have my HIV consultant to thank for putting me in touch with good immigration specialists when I was first diagnosed and THT and George House Trust have also provided very good support.

Nor can I forget the support I have received from other people with HIV in the UK - and they haven't all been Africans! It has been wonderful.

But there has been discrimination and stigma. When I was first dispersed to Manchester, somebody I had to share with searched through my bags and found letters saying I had HIV. This person told other people I shared with and they asked me how I got infected with HIV. The worst thing is when you experience stigma from other people who have HIV.

Thanks to George House Trust I was moved and have my own place where I know my daughter and I are safe. But I still do worry - what will happen to me if we were sent back to Zimbabwe and I cannot get anti-HIV drugs? Thankfully I have sisters and I know that they will bring up my child if I die.

My experiences have taught me that it is really important not to give up hope when you find out you have HIV. Knowing that you have HIV means that you can start seeing a doctor who can help stop you becoming ill. Also, it's important to get help as soon as possible over immigration problems - don't ignore these problems if they come up as they will not go away.

So I'll finish by saying, when you find out you are HIV-positive, try and keep up a positive attitude, it really made a difference for me.

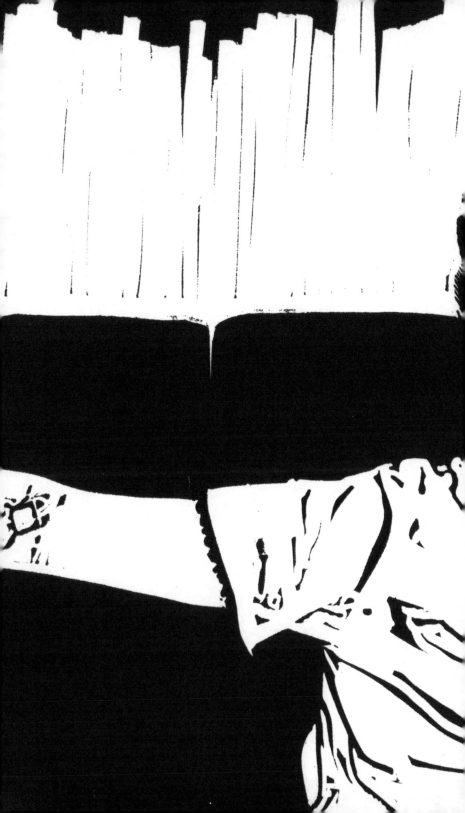

Key tests to monitor HIV

CD4 and viral load

In this chapter you'll find information on

The importance of tests to assess how HIV is affecting you.

CD4 cell counts, a key test used to assess the health of the immune system that is used to help guide decisions about when to start HIV treatment and to monitor how effective HIV treatment is.

Viral load tests, which measure the amount of HIV in the blood and are used along with CD4 cell counts to decide when to start HIV treatment and to see if your HIV treatment is working.

An explanation of what an 'undetectable' viral load is.

Other blood tests to monitor your health.

Why monitor?

There are two key tests that doctors use to assess how HIV is affecting your body.

The CD4 cell count is a guide to how strong your immune system is. The viral load test measures the amount of HIV in your blood.

Regular monitoring of CD4 cell count and HIV viral load provide a good indication of the effects of HIV on your body. Doctors can interpret your test results in the context of what they know about the course of HIV disease progression.

For example, your risk of developing opportunistic infections is directly related to your CD4 cell count - PCP pneumonia rarely occurs in people whose CD4 cell count is above 200 - 250. The level of your viral load predicts how rapidly your CD4 cell count is likely to fall. When looked at together, these two results can be used to predict your risk of developing AIDS in the next few years. For example, if your HIV viral load is above 55,000 and your CD4 cell count below 200, then there's an 85% chance that you'll develop AIDS in the next three years. This is illustrated in the table on the next page.

Results from your CD4 cell count and viral load tests can help you and your doctor make decisions about when to take HIV treatments, or therapy to help prevent you from developing opportunistic infections.

CD4 cell counts
What CD4 cells do
CD4 cells, sometimes also called T-cells, or T-helper cells, are white blood cells which organise the immune system's response to bacterial, fungal and viral infections.

CD4 cell counts in people without HIV
A normal CD4 cell count in an HIV-negative man is between 400 and 1600 per cubic millimetre of blood. CD4 cell counts in HIV-negative women tend to be a little higher, between 500 - 1600.

Predicting progression

% of people who develop AIDS within 3 years (assuming no treatment)

Viral load	CD4				
	below 200	201-350	351-500	501-750	above 750
below 1,500	**	**	**	3.7	0
1,500-7,000	**	**	2.0	2.0	2.0
7,000-20,000	**	8.1	8.1	8.1	3.2
20,000-55,000	40.1	40.1	16.1	16.1	9.5
above 55,000	85.5	64.4	42.9	32.6	32.6

** indicates lack of data

Even if you don't have HIV, many factors can affect your CD4 cell count. For example it's known that:

- Women have higher CD4 cell counts than men (by about 100).

- Women's CD4 cell counts go up and down during the menstrual cycle.

- Oral contraceptives can lower a woman's CD4 cell count.

- Smokers tend to have higher CD4 cell counts (by about 140).

- CD4 cell counts fall after rest - by as much as 40%.

- A good night's sleep can mean that you have a lower CD4 cell count the following morning, but a higher CD4 cell count the next afternoon.

None of these factors seems to make any difference to how able your immune system is to fight infections.

Only a small portion of your body's CD4 cells are in the blood. The rest are in the lymph nodes and tissue, and the fluctuations noted above might be due to the movement of CD4 cells between blood and tissue.

CD4 cell counts in people with HIV

Soon after infection with HIV, your CD4 cell count probably dropped sharply, before stabilising at around 500 - 600. It seems that people who experience a greater initial drop in CD4 cell count and a lower stabilisation in their CD4 cell count may be at risk of faster disease progression. Even while you are well and have no obvious symptoms of HIV, millions of CD4 cells are infected by HIV and lost every day, and millions more are produced to replace them.

It's estimated, however, that without treatment, an HIV-positive person's CD4 cell count drops by about 45 cells every six months, with greater falls experienced by people with higher CD4 cell counts.

A CD4 cell count between 200 and 500 indicates that some damage to your immune system has occurred.

Steeper falls in CD4 cell counts are experienced in the year before AIDS develops, which is why you are recommended to have your CD4 cell count regularly monitored once it goes below 350.

Looking at your CD4 cell count can also provide a guide for decisions about your need to take medicines to prevent some AIDS-defining illnesses. For example, if your CD4 cell count is below 200, you are recommended to take antibiotics to prevent you getting PCP pneumonia.

Your CD4 cell count can naturally fluctuate, so don't put too much emphasis on a single test result. Rather, look at the trend in a number of recent CD4 cell counts.

If your CD4 cell count is high, you have no symptoms, and are not taking anti-HIV medication, then it probably only needs monitoring every few months or so.

However, if it's falling rapidly, you are unwell, are taking part in a clinical trial, or are taking anti-HIV drugs, then it should be monitored more often.

CD4 cell percentages
Sometimes, as well as counting the number of CD4 cells, doctors will also assess what percentage of all your white blood cells are CD4 cells. This is called the CD4 cell percentage. A normal result in a person with an intact immune system is about 40%, and a CD4 cell percentage below 20% indicates the same risk of becoming ill with an AIDS-defining illness as a CD4 cell count of about 200.

CD4 cell counts and HIV treatment
Your CD4 cell count can be used to help decide when you need to start anti-HIV treatment, and as an indication of how successful these treatments are.

Once your CD4 cell falls to about 350, your doctor should start talking to you about whether you need to start taking anti-HIV treatments.

If your CD4 cell count falls to between 200 and 250 cells, you are recommended to start anti-HIV treatment. A CD4 cell count of this level indicates that you are at a real risk of becoming ill with an AIDS-defining illness.

It also seems that if you wait until your CD4 cell count falls to below 200, you are less likely to respond well to anti-HIV treatment. However, there doesn't seem to be any health benefit from starting HIV treatment if your CD4 cell count is above 350.

Once you start anti-HIV treatment, your CD4 cell count should start to slowly increase. If you experience a fall in your CD4 cell count over a number of tests, this should alert your doctor that there's something wrong with your HIV treatments.

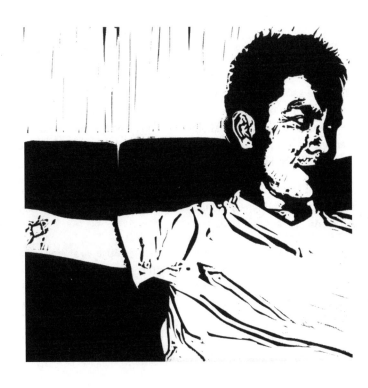

Viral load

What is viral load?

Viral load is the amount of HIV in the blood.

The more HIV you have in your blood, the faster your CD4 cell count will fall, and the greater your risk of developing symptoms of HIV infection or AIDS-defining illnesses.

People taking anti-HIV drugs normally see an increase in their CD4 cell count as viral load falls. If you're taking treatment, monitoring your viral load gives an indication of how well your treatments are working.

What is the viral load test?

Viral load tests estimate the number of HIV particles circulating in the liquid, or plasma, part of the blood. They do this by looking for HIV's genes, which are called HIV RNA.

The result of a viral load test is described as the number of copies of HIV RNA per millilitre. For example, a viral load of two hundred would be written as 200 copies/ml. But your doctor is likely to describe your viral load using just the number.

There are several different viral load tests, or assays, in use at the moment. These tests use different techniques to measure the number of HIV particles, but the tests are equally reliable at showing whether your viral load is low, medium, or high. The PCR (polymerase chain reaction) assay is the one most commonly used in the UK.

Viral load tests used in this country are equally accurate at measuring types of HIV (called subtypes) found in other parts of the world, for example Africa and Asia.

It's now usual to use what are called ultra-sensitive viral load tests. These are able to detect viral load as low as 50 copies/ml. If your viral load is below 50 copies/ml, it is said to be 'undetectable' and, for most people, getting an undetectable viral load is one of the key goals of anti-HIV treatment. It's important to remember however, having an undetectable viral load doesn't mean that you have been cured of HIV. This is considered in a lot more detail in the chapter *Anti-HIV treatment.*

Understanding your viral load results

A viral load above 100,000 copies/ml is considered high, and one below 10,000 copies/ml is considered low.

But your viral load can seem to fluctuate quite widely from one test to another if you are not on treatment, even though this has no implications for your health.

Indeed, doctors have looked at viral load changes in people not on anti-HIV treatment and have found that two separate tests on the same sample of blood can give widely different results. So you shouldn't get too worried if your viral load increases from 5,000 copies/ml to 15,000 copies/ml when you're not on treatment. Even an increase from 50,000 copies/ml to 100,000 copies/ml isn't necessarily that important if you're not on treatment. Although it appears that your viral load might have doubled, it's within the margin of error for the test.

Rather than attaching too much importance to a single viral load test result, look at the trend in your viral load over time. The time of day your blood sample is taken could influence your viral load, and your viral load might temporarily increase if you're unwell with an infection before falling back again. Similarly, some vaccinations can cause a temporary variation in your viral load.

You should, however, be concerned if your viral load results over several months show an upward trend, or if the increase is greater than threefold. For example, an increase from 5,000 to 15,000 isn't significant, but an increase from 5,000 to 25,000 is.

Undetectable viral load

All viral load tests have a cut-off point below which they cannot reliably detect HIV. This is called the limit of detection, and the tests used in the UK have a lower limit of detection of 50 copies/ml. If your viral load is below 50 it is said to be undetectable.

But just because the level of HIV is too low to be measured doesn't mean that HIV has disappeared from your blood. It might still be present in the blood, but in amounts too low to be measured. As viral load tests only measure levels of HIV in the blood, the viral load in other parts of your body, for example your lymph nodes or sexual fluids, might be detectable.

Why it's good to have an undetectable viral load

Having an undetectable viral load is desirable for two reasons. It means that you are at a very low risk of becoming ill because of HIV, and also that there is a very low risk that you will become resistant to your anti-HIV treatments.

HIV can only become resistant to a drug if it continues to reproduce whilst you are taking that drug. If the reproduction of HIV is kept at very low levels, the appearance of drug resistance should be delayed, perhaps indefinitely. This means that your anti-HIV drugs go on working.

Because of this, HIV doctors now stress that an aim of anti-HIV treatment should be to get HIV viral load down to undetectable levels as soon as possible, ideally within six months of starting HIV treatment.

Some people take three to six months to reach this point, others go below detection within four to twelve weeks, and others may never reach this goal.

For a discussion on whether people who have an undetectable viral load are infectious, see the section *Sex and HIV*.

Viral load blips

If your viral load is undetectable, there's a good chance that your viral load might occasionally increase above 50 copies/ml to 100 or 200 copies/ml in a single test before falling back to being undetectable. These are called viral load blips and they do not indicate that your anti-HIV treatment is failing. Indeed, most blips seem to be due to testing errors at the laboratory.

Viral load in women

Women seem to have lower viral loads than men with the same CD4 cell counts. This doesn't have any effect on the rate of HIV disease progression and the reasons for it aren't properly understood. It's been suggested that women might have lower viral loads due to a superior immune response to infections; or that viral production is naturally lower in women.

Looking at CD4 and viral load together

If you're not currently taking anti-HIV treatment

If you're not currently taking anti-HIV treatment, your viral load and CD4 cell count can help predict your risk of becoming ill because of HIV in the future.

Among people with the same CD4 cell counts, research has shown that those with a higher viral load tend to develop symptoms more quickly than those with a lower viral load.

In addition, among people with the same viral load, those with lower CD4 cell counts tend to become ill more quickly.

As the table in the section 'Why monitor?' earlier in this chapter shows, looked at together, your CD4 cell count and viral load provide an indication of your risk of developing AIDS in the short to medium term.

For example, if you look at the column for people with a CD4 cell count between 351 and 500 you can see that there is a big variation in the risk of disease progression, depending on the level of viral load.

Deciding when to start treatment

Your viral load and CD4 cell count can help you decide if you need to start taking anti-HIV treatment.

At the moment, doctors put more emphasis on the level of your CD4 cell count, and it is recommended that you start treatment before your CD4 cell count falls below 200. This is because your risk of death is greater if you start treatment when your CD4 cell count is below 200.

At higher CD4 cell counts, the picture is much less clear, and your decision will depend on a combination of the level of your viral load, the speed at which your CD4 cell count is falling, any symptoms you may have, and your wishes.

The question of when to start HIV treatment is looked at in a lot more detail in the chapter *Anti-HIV treatment*.

Monitoring the effectiveness of treatment

Effective anti-HIV treatment results in a fall in your viral load. Within about four weeks of starting HIV treatment, your doctor should test your viral load to see how much it has fallen.

The aim of treatment in people who have never taken anti-HIV drugs before is to get viral load to undetectable levels within 24 weeks.

As your viral load falls, your CD4 cell count should begin to slowly increase.

Frequency of testing

If you're not on treatment

Even if your CD4 cell count is above 500, it's a good idea to go to your HIV clinic every three to six months for a CD4 cell count and viral load test. Make sure you go back promptly for your results.

If your CD4 cell count is between 200 and 350, you'll need to go to your clinic every couple of months, or even monthly, to have your CD4 cell count and viral load checked.

If you're about to start treatment

You should be given a 'baseline' CD4 cell count and two viral load measurements close together shortly before starting treatment. You and your doctors will then be able to assess how effective your treatment has been, by looking at how much your viral load has fallen and your CD4 cell count has risen.

If you're on treatment

You should have your viral load and CD4 cell count measured a month after starting treatment and then about three months after that.

Subsequent CD4 cell counts and viral load tests should be carried out every ten to twelve weeks. Additional tests might be needed if you feel unwell or develop symptoms.

If your viral load increases whilst you are on treatment, you should have a further test within a week or two to confirm this, and your CD4 cell count should be monitored at the same time to see if there's been a fall.

Other tests

As well as monitoring your CD4 cell count and viral load, it's highly likely that you'll have other blood tests as well. Details of the some of the tests you can expect to have are provided below.

Blood counts

Doctors conduct blood counts to see if you are at risk of anaemia (a shortage of red blood cells).

Anaemia can be caused as a result of HIV disease itself. The nucleoside reverse transcriptase inhibitor (NRTI) AZT (zidovudine, *Retrovir*) and any combination pill that contains AZT (*Combivir* or *Trizivir*) can cause anaemia. The protease inhibitor indinavir (*Crixivan*) has been linked to a small number of cases of anaemia.

Liver function tests
It's very likely that you'll have regular blood tests to monitor the function of your liver.

The non-nucleoside analogue nevirapine (*Viramune*) can be toxic to the liver, as can protease inhibitors. Medicines used to treat other infections that people with HIV are vulnerable to can also cause liver problems.

Your doctor is likely to monitor your liver particularly closely if you are also infected with hepatitis B virus or hepatitis C virus (serious viruses which affect the liver).

Many people with HIV only discovered that they were infected with either (or both) hepatitis B or C because they had an abnormal liver function test result and were tested for the presence of these viruses.

Liver function tests look for levels of proteins in the blood, including serum albumin and bilirubin. Other liver function tests include assessing alanine aminotransferase (ALT) and aspartate aminotransferase (AST).

Metabolic tests
Levels of cholesterol (fats) in the blood can be disturbed by anti-HIV drugs, particularly protease inhibitors.Cholesterol, triglycerides, blood sugars, and glucose can also be affected by HIV drugs. You are likely to have tests to monitor the level of your cholesterol, triglycerides and glucose just before you start anti-HIV drugs and then again every time you attend the clinic thereafter.

Liver function tests can give an indication if you have the rare but very serious side-effect lactic acidosis. This can be caused by some drugs in the NRTI class.

Blood samples may also be measured to check levels of the enzyme amylase. Abnormal levels of amylase can be a warning sign that you are at risk of the very serious side-effect pancreatitis. This can be caused by some NRTI drugs.

Kidney function test

Tests will also be conducted to see how well your kidneys are working, particularly if you are taking the protease inhibitor indinavir (*Crixivan*) or the nucleotide analogue tenofovir (*Viread*), as both these drugs are known to cause kidney problems.

Syphilis

If you are sexually active with more than one partner, your clinic may well test you regularly for syphilis. Recent outbreaks of syphilis in several cities in the UK, Europe, and American have been focused on HIV-positive gay men.

Further reading

- NAM factsheet, *CD4 T-cell counts, Immune system cells, Liver function tests* and *Viral load*.

- *CD4 and viral load*, booklet produced by NAM.

- 'Viral load, CD4 cell counts and other tests' in NAM's *HIV and AIDS Treatments Directory*.

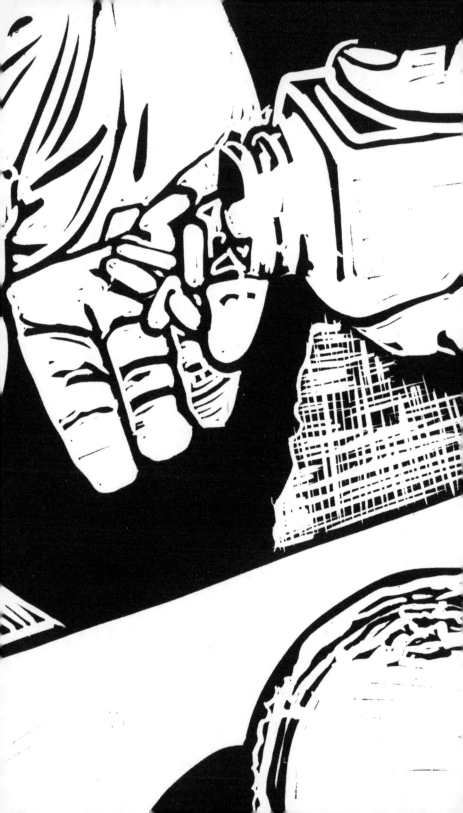

Anti-HIV treatment

In this chapter you'll find information on

When anti-HIV treatment should
be started.

The names of the different anti-HIV drugs.

Which drugs are recommended for first-line
HIV treatment.

Some questions you might want to ask your
doctor before starting treatment.

When and why you may want to change
HIV treatment.

What options are available for people who
have taken a lot of anti-HIV drugs.

Treatment breaks.

There are five first-hand accounts of life on
anti-HIV treatment, four by men and one by
an anonymous author.

Treatment, not a cure

There is no cure for HIV. However, when taken properly, combinations of different antiretroviral drugs can reduce the amount of HIV in the blood to levels so low that they cannot be detected using the tests that we currently have.

Reducing the amount of HIV, or HIV viral load, has been shown to reduce the risk of becoming ill or dying because of HIV. So, reducing HIV viral load, and keeping it low, is the aim of anti-HIV treatment.

In the UK and the US, the aim of HIV treatment for people who have never taken HIV drugs before and most other people with experience of HIV treatment is to get and maintain an undetectable viral load - i.e. a viral load below 50, the cut-off point for the ultrasensitive tests in routine use.

As your HIV viral load goes down, your immune system will start to recover. This should be indicated by an increase in your CD4 cell count, and there's also a good chance that you'll notice an improvement in your health at the same time, if you have been ill due to HIV.

If you have taken lots of HIV drugs, and still have a detectable viral load, then the aim of your treatment might be to boost your CD4 cell count to protect you from infections rather than to achieve an undetectable viral load. But as anti-HIV drugs have got better, doctors are now hopeful that they can get an undetectable viral load in people who have take a lot of HIV drugs before.

Some researchers have looked at whether treatment with anti-HIV drugs can eliminate, or eradicate, HIV from the body. It was thought by some doctors that treatment during the very early stages of HIV might offer the best chance of achieving this. But even though treatment with powerful combinations of anti-HIV drugs can be successful at getting viral load down to very low levels, HIV will still infect cells and reproduce itself at those very low levels. Anti-HIV drugs can't kill these cells. This means that, with the currently available drugs, eradication of HIV is not possible.

Even when HIV is being suppressed to undetectable low levels, the remaining virus could rebound to high levels if you stop taking your anti-HIV drugs. What's more, anti-HIV drugs are less good at controlling HIV replication in the brain, and other organs of the body.

When to start treatment

It's not known for certain what is the best time to start treatment with anti-HIV drugs. This means you need to weigh up with your doctor, on an individual basis, the likely benefits and risks of starting treatment now as opposed to waiting until later.

However, it's currently recommended in UK HIV treatment guidelines that you start anti-HIV treatments immediately if you are ill because of HIV, or have an AIDS-defining illness. It's also recommended that you start treatment if your CD4 cell count is near or below 200, the level at which you become vulnerable to serious AIDS-defining illnesses, or is falling very rapidly.

UK treatment guidelines also make other recommendations about whether you should take HIV treatments, depending on the length of time you have been infected with HIV, the level of your CD4 cell count and the amount of HIV in your blood - your viral load.

Recently infected with HIV?

The six months after you are infected by HIV is called primary HIV infection. There is no proof that taking treatment at this time will mean that you live a longer, healthier life. Some doctors believe, however, that treatment at this time may offer a unique chance to control HIV which may be lost later, as your immune system sustains ongoing damage due to HIV, and becomes less able to attack HIV. Whatever your CD4 cell count, if you are considering treatment soon after infection, you should start as soon as possible, and certainly within six months of infection with HIV. Clinical trials are underway to assess the effectiveness of taking anti-HIV treatment at this stage and you might wish to consider joining one.

The potential benefits of taking treatment at this time need to be weighed up against the risk of side-effects. Treatments may reduce your quality of life at a time when HIV would not have. There is also a possibility that if your treatments don't work effectively against HIV, drug resistance could develop, and you would have fewer drug options if you became ill because of HIV.

A very small number of people become really quite ill during primary infection with HIV, and might even need to be admitted to hospital. Taking anti-HIV treatment at this stage may be particularly beneficial in these circumstances. But it's not clear how long you'll need to take treatment for - current practice is to treat for six months to a year - and you might experience symptoms again once you stop your treatment.

Infected with HIV for over six months, but without symptoms?

Ideally, you should begin treatment before your CD4 count falls below 200. This is because if you start treatment when your CD4 count is below 200, you face a greater risk of ill health and even death, in the short term, than if you start while your CD4 count is still above 200.

At higher CD4 counts, the picture is less clear. Most studies suggest that there seems to be no difference in the short-term risk of ill health if you begin treatment at CD4 counts above the 200 level. Therefore, the timing in these circumstances will depend on the level of your viral load, the speed at which your CD4 count is falling, the likelihood of you achieving good adherence to treatment, the presence of symptoms, the presence of hepatitis C virus coinfection and your wishes.

You may choose an earlier start, particularly if your CD4 count is falling by more than 80 cells per year, because this is likely to mean that the count will fall below 200 within the near future. Similarly, if you have a high viral load, and are not taking treatment, then you lose CD4 cells more quickly than others, and are at greater risk of illness or death in the short term, and you may, therefore, choose to start treatment sooner.

You may wish to consider starting treatment earlier if you are also infected with hepatitis C virus, as liver disease becomes worse when the CD4 cell count is lower. There's a lot more information on hepatitis C in the section 'Illness in the age of anti-HIV treatment - hepatitis.'

Delaying therapy reduces the impact of long-term side-effects and the development of drug resistance. Therapies of the future may be easier to take, less toxic and perhaps more effective against HIV. The best responses to anti-HIV treatment are generally seen with the first drug combination, so starting too early, or with the wrong drug combination may not be the best option.

If you are advised to start treatment but choose not to, then you should review your decision regularly and have your CD4 count and viral load monitored more frequently than usually recommended, for example every two months.

Infected with HIV for over six months, and ill because of HIV?

Regardless of your CD4 cell count, doctors recommend that you should take anti-HIV treatments if you are becoming ill because of HIV.

A possible exception, however, would be if you have tuberculosis. There are potential interactions between anti-HIV drugs and a key medicine used to treat tuberculosis. Because of this, many doctors recommend delaying treatment with anti-HIV drugs until a person has taken at least two months of tuberculosis treatment. Similarly, if you become ill with tuberculosis whilst taking HIV treatment, you may be recommended to stop taking anti-HIV drugs for the first two months of tuberculosis treatment.

If your CD4 cell count is below 200 you should start anti-HIV treatment immediately.

Starting anti-HIV treatment

Most people who are taking anti-HIV drugs will take a combination, or 'regimen', of three drugs. There are exceptions to this, for example pregnant women (see the chapter *Symptoms and illnesses*), or those who have a very high viral load and need to take more than three drugs to obtain a powerful anti-HIV effect.

Before you start HIV treatment for the first time you should have a test to see if you were infected with a strain of HIV with resistance to anti-HIV drugs.

Anti-HIV drug classes and names

There are currently 19 drugs licensed and used for the treatment of HIV, and these drugs are divided into one of four classes depending on how they attack HIV.

Listed below are the classes of drug and the individual drugs within each class. Anti-HIV drugs tend to have more than one name. Listed first is the name the drug is normally called by in this country, then in brackets the generic name for the drug is listed, and finally the drug company's patented tradename for the drug.

Nucleoside/nucleotide reverse transcriptase inhibitors (NRTI, or Nukes for short)

Drugs in this class include AZT (zidovudine, *Retrovir*),ddI (didanosine, *Videx*), 3TC (lamivudine, *Epivir*), d4T (stavudine, *Zerit*), abacavir (*Ziagen*), and FTC (emtricitabine, *Emtriva*). There is also a nucleotide analogue reverse transcriptase inhibitor called tenofovir (*Viread*).

AZT and 3TC is available in a combined pill called *Combivir* and AZT, 3TC and abacavir is available in a combined pill called *Trizivir*.

There is also a single pill combining AZT and abacavir, called *Kivexa*.

A single pill combining FTC and the nucleotide analogue tenofovir called *Truvada* is a also available.

Non-nucleoside reverse transcriptase inhibitors (NNRTI, or non-Nukes for short)
Drugs in this class are efavirenz (*Sustiva*) and nevirapine (*Viramune*).

Protease inhibitors (PIs)
Drugs in this class are lopinavir/ritonavir (*Kaletra*), indinavir (*Crixivan*), ritonavir (*Norvir*), nelfinavir (*Viracept*), saquinavir hard gel capsules (*Invirase*), atazanavir (*Reyataz*), amprenavir (*Agenerase*), fosamprenavir (*Telzir*), tipranavir (*Aptivus*).

Fusion inhibitor
There is only one drug available in this class, T20 (enfuvirtide, *Fuzeon*).

Finding out more
You can find out a lot more about these drugs including by visiting www.aidsmap.com, or by reading the NAM booklet *Anti-HIV drugs*, which is available free of charge from HIV clinics, or can be downloaded from aidsmap.com.

First combination

NNRTI-based
An NNRTI should be taken with a combination of two nucleoside/nucleotide reverse transcriptase inhibitors (NRTIs). Either:

- tenofovir/FTC (available in a combination pill, *Truvada*)

- abacavir/3TC (available in a combination pill, *Kivexa*)

- AZT/3TC (available in a combination pill, *Combivir*)

However, AZT has been associated with body shape changes and your doctor should discuss the risks of these occurring, and side-effects which abacavir and tenofovir can cause, before you decide which drugs to take.

The reason why some doctors and people with HIV often prefer an NNRTI-based combination is that it has relatively few side-effects and is very easy to take. However, it is very easy to develop resistance to NNRTIs, and if you become resistant to one it's unlikely you'll benefit from using any of the currently available NNRTIs.

Protease inhibitor-based

Boosted protease inhibitors include a small dose of the protease inhibitor ritonavir (*Norvir*). If you choose to take a boosted protease inhibitor it is likely that your doctor will recommend that you take *Kaletra* (lopinavir/ritonavir). Other options are fosamprenavir/ritonavir (*Telzir*) and hard gel saquinavir/ritonavir (*Invirase*). At the moment, there is not enough evidence for atazanavir/ritonavir (*Reyataz*) to be recommend for first-line treatment.

You can also take a first anti-HIV combination that is based on protease inhibitors. However, if you do take a protease inhibitor as part of your first treatment regimen, it should be a 'boosted' protease inhibitor. The addition of the small dose of ritonavir boosts blood levels of the drug, meaning that it has a more powerful anti-HIV effect and you have to take fewer pills, which might make your combination easier to adhere to.

Most British doctors think that it is probably best to start with a combination that involves a non-nucleoside reverse transcriptase inhibitor (NNRTI), or a boosted protease inhibitor.

Which nucleotides/nucleotide?

Anti-HIV treatment regimens almost always include two nucleoside/nucleotide analogues. It's not really known which two provide the most effective combination. However, you shouldn't take d4T in your first anti-HIV drug combination because of concerns about side-effects. There are also concerns about the possible side-effects of AZT and your doctor should discuss these, and the side-effects caused by all other drugs in the nucleoside/nucleotide class before you reach a decision about which drugs to take.

The nucleotide analogue tenofovir has been successfully used in initial combinations, and your doctor may be particularly likely to prescribe it if you are infected with hepatitis B virus as well as HIV, when it should be prescribed with 3TC or FTC which is also effective against hepatitis B. You should not take ddI and tenofovir together because the drugs interact unless you have no other options available to you.

HIV medicine is evolving very quickly. You can get regular updates on HIV treatments and the best ways to use them by visiting www.aidsmap.com. You can also get a free subscription to *AIDS Treatment Update* (ATU), NAM's monthly treatments newsletter, by filling in the form at the back of this book and returning it to the freepost address.

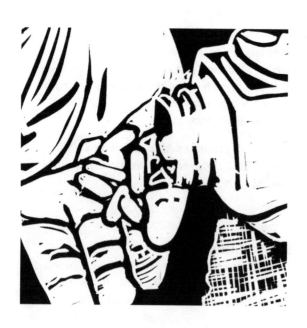

Questions to ask your doctor before starting treatment

What's in the name of a drug?

All medications have at least two names: a generic one, such as zidovudine, and a trade name, such as *Retrovir*, which is used to market the drug and which appears prominently on the packaging, and sometimes on the capsule or tablet itself. Some are also referred to using an abbreviation of their chemical name, e.g. AZT. It is useful to be familiar with all of these names

What does it look like?

If you are trying to decide what medication to take, it may be useful to see the tablets you will have to take. Some people have more difficulty swallowing large pills than others, and if you think the tablets are very large this may cause you difficulties taking them in the future.

The free booklet called *Anti-HIV Drugs* produced by NAM includes pictures of all the drugs and details of the doses, and brief answers to all of the following questions for each drug currently prescribed.

How and when do I need to take it?

Regimens vary from once to four or more times a day, and you may be keen to minimise the number of times you have to take medication each day. Once- or twice-daily dosing is generally found easier to live with than more frequent dosing. For more information on taking anti-HIV drugs see the chapter *Adherence*.

What side-effects might I experience?

Most drugs will have side-effects, especially during the first few weeks of treatment. If you know what to expect you may find them easier to deal with, or you may decide that you will find a particular type of side-effect particularly bothersome, and would therefore prefer to avoid it. Each drug is associated with different side-effects, but the most common early side-effects tend to be:

- nausea
- headache
- rash
- vomiting
- diarrhoea
- fatigue

Other side-effects may emerge later and may only show up on blood tests, for example:

- tingling in the hands and feet leading to eventual nerve damage (peripheral neuropathy)
- liver toxicities
- neutropenia (low levels of white blood cells needed to fight infections)
- anaemia (low levels of oxygen-bearing red blood cells, leading to tiredness)
- lipodystrophy (changes in body fat) - either fat loss from the face and limbs or fat accumulation in the abdomen and breasts.

Many other side-effects may appear in very small numbers of people. For example, a small number of people who have taken protease inhibitors have experienced the onset of diabetes. Because anti-HIV drugs are only tested in a few thousand people before being licensed for widespread use, there is a chance that very rare side-effects will only become apparent when tens of thousands of people have taken the drug.

For more information see the chapter *Side-effects.*

When are the side-effects likely to happen?

Most drug side-effects happen in the first few weeks of treatment as the body adjusts to processing the drug. After a few weeks they begin to get better. Many people report considerable fatigue during the first months of treatment, but it is not clear why this is so.

For more information, see the chapter *Side-effects.*

What can I do to relieve any side-effects I experience?

It is often possible to relieve side-effects by taking other medication which will not interfere with your anti-HIV therapy. For example, your doctor can prescribe anti-nausea drugs and anti-diarrhoea drugs, and painkillers can be used to relieve headaches. Some rashes can be relieved by antihistamines or perhaps steroids, and taking the drugs with food (if recommended) may reduce nausea. However, nothing has yet been discovered to combat the fatigue that may accompany the early stages of a new anti-retroviral regimen, so the only remedy for this is to rest until your energy returns.

Another option with some drugs is to increase the dose gradually.

Is it okay to stop treatment if I can't stand the side-effects, or want a break?

It is best to consult with your doctor before making any changes. You should bear in mind that stopping a drug for more than a few days may mean that you will experience the same side-effects all over again if you resume treatment. Similarly, any gains made in terms of lowering your viral load or raising your CD4 count may be lost quickly whilst you are off treatment.

If you miss doses or reduce the dose rather than stopping treatment altogether, you are likely to increase your risk of developing resistance to one or more of the drugs you are taking (and, potentially, cross-resistance to related drugs that you have not yet taken). However, this varies according to the drugs you are taking. Some drugs leave the body more slowly than others, which is another reason to speak to your doctor beforehand.

Structured treatment interruptions, (the scientific name for treatment breaks) are being investigated by researchers as a means of controlling HIV. However, whether their benefits may outweigh their risks is not yet established. In the meantime, experts have agreed that it is not safe for individuals to experiment with their treatment in this way, unless it is part of a clinical trial.

What can I do if I miss a dose or take too much?

If you miss a single dose by a few hours you should take the missed dose as soon as you can and take the next dose at the normal time. However, if you have missed the dose completely, and only realise this when you come to take the next dose, there is no additional benefit in taking a double dose.

Missed doses are problematic because they lead to falls in drug levels. In turn this can encourage the development of resistance. Missing doses regularly (for example, every weekend) will probably encourage the development of resistance. On the other hand, the occasional missed dose may not cause too many problems.

You may wish to experiment before you start an antiretroviral regimen to see that you can manage it. Try and make it as realistic as possible. If you have several different sorts of low dose vitamin tablets this will be a harmless way of modelling the practice of taking three different drugs at set times each day. Try this for a month and see how you get on. This is a painless way of testing whether you can adhere to a regimen successfully. If you can't manage the regimen you've tested in this way, you may be best advised to look for another one which suits you better.

If you've taken other medication for non-HIV related problems before, don't assume that these will predict your likely adherence to combination therapy. Any medication which prevents the immediate recurrence of a condition is likely to be taken more consistently than one where the effect of non-compliance is only visible through laboratory tests.

For more information see the chapter *Adherence*.

Will anti-HIV drugs interact with other drugs I take?

Anti-HIV drugs, particularly protease inhibitors, interact with many other drugs including prescription drugs, over-the-counter drugs, recreational drugs and herbal preparations. Drug interactions may cause serious side-effects. Furthermore, interactions may mean that one or more of your medicines don't work properly.

Do I need to take the drugs on a full or empty stomach?

The absorption of some drugs can be seriously affected by the presence of absence of food in the stomach. For these drugs you will be instructed to take your medication with or without food as necessary.

Are there any foods I should avoid?

You should be given detailed instructions about what you should and shouldn't eat when taking this medication. Fortunately, the restrictions on food relate more to whether you should take drugs on a full stomach or not rather than whether you should avoid food.

Do I need to be careful about drinking or recreational drug use on this treatment?

Very few anti-HIV drugs are affected by alcohol, although the pancreatitis risk of some drugs, such as ddI, may be increased if you drink heavily, in the view of some doctors. Pancreatitis and peripheral neuropathy are in any case associated with heavy alcohol consumption. Alcohol may also affect your liver's capacity to process antiretroviral drugs, and may increase nausea.

For information about anti-HIV drugs and recreational drugs see the chapter *Daily health issues*.

What do I do if I think I am pregnant or want to become pregnant?

If you are already on treatment, any potential adverse effects of drugs on your baby are most likely to occur during the first 14 weeks of pregnancy. HIV transmission is more likely to occur during delivery, but transmission has been shown to occur during the first 14 weeks of pregnancy, so the option of stopping treatment needs to be balanced against the potential risk of a rebound in viral load if you come off treatment. Increased viral load increases the risk of HIV transmission from mother to child.

If you want to conceive you should discuss the relative risks of coming off treatment or conceiving whilst on treatment with your doctor.

For more information see *Mother-to-baby transmission of HIV*.

Do I need to think about taking time off work while my body gets used to these drugs?

Some people find that it may take several weeks before they feel well enough to go back to work, or before they can manage without childcare assistance, when they begin anti-HIV treatment.

Do these drugs need to be kept in the fridge or in a special container?

Some drugs may deteriorate in hot conditions and so may require refrigeration, or to be stored in a cool place, out of direct sunlight. Other drugs, for example indinavir, may be affected by damp conditions. This drug must be kept in a container with a special dessicant (a substance which draws moisture out of the air) and shouldn't be kept in a box with other pills, or in the fridge. Your doctor or pharmacist will be able to provide advice on this.

Can I take them on holiday?

The major difficulty with taking these drugs on holiday is the number of containers you may have to carry and the attention this may draw to your HIV-positive status. However, none of the packaging for these drugs reveals that they are prescribed for the treatment of HIV infection, and a letter from your doctor which says that you are prescribed these specific drugs should provide sufficient cover for you. Difficulty may come for people who wish to enter the United States however, where entry for HIV-positive people is restricted.

If you are going to a hot climate lopinavir, ritonavir and saquinavir may deteriorate because of the heat, and indinavir may deteriorate because of humidity. Be sure to keep indinavir capsules in a dry place, and keep them in the original container with the dessicant supplied as far as possible.

Alterations in time zones and the eating schedules (and size of portions!) on long-haul flights may be more problematic. People who work on airlines tend to keep to the time zone of their home country wherever they are working, but this is more difficult for people who are travelling somewhere for several days or weeks. Although airlines recommend that you switch into the time zone of your destination as soon as the flight begins (in order to combat jet lag), this may be confusing if you are trying to stick to a schedule. Eight- or twelve-hour changes in time zones are likely to be relatively easy to work with; shorter or longer adjustments (from Europe to the Middle East, Latin America, the East Coast of the United States, India, Australia and the Pacific) may be more problematic.

If you are gone for less than five days, it will probably work out easier to stick to home time, but if you are away for longer, try to tailor your dosing times to the time zone of your destination as quickly as possible without missing doses (remember that with most drugs you have a couple of hours leeway either side of the twelve-hour or eight-hour intervals at which you are meant to take the drugs).

For more information see the chapters *Adherence* and *Travel*.

Should I drive a car or operate machinery while taking these drugs?
If any medication is causing drowsiness, dizziness, loss of concentration or fatigue, you should be very careful about driving or operating machinery. These have all been reported as early side-effects of some antiretroviral drugs.

How can I get further information about this treatment?
A variety of sources can provide you with information about the treatment prescribed to you, but at the very least your doctor should provide you with a clear explanation of any of the issues discussed in this section, supported by written information to take home. Some drug companies have produced information booklets about their drugs which may answer some of these questions, but if your doctor is not available, the first port of call may be your HIV pharmacist, who should know the answers to all the questions discussed in this section. Your doctor should provide you with information on where to go if you have any questions on your treatment.

Changing treatment due to failure

As mentioned above, the goal of anti-HIV treatment, if you are taking it for the first time, is to reduce your viral load to below the limit of detection, which, using current tests, is 50 copies/ml. If your viral load doesn't fall below this level, then it's more likely that your treatments won't suppress HIV for long.

If your viral load falls below 50, then rebounds to above 50 on two consecutive tests, then it means that your treatment is failing. You may find that your CD4 cell count starts to fall, which will mean that your risk of becoming ill because of HIV increases.

If your treatment fails to get your viral load below 50, or it rebounds above this level, then there's a possible risk that you will develop resistance to some or all of the anti-HIV drugs you are taking.

If your treatment is not suppressing your viral load to undetectable levels, it should be changed.

Occasionally, your viral load may rise a little above 50 before dropping down to undetectable levels on the next test. These changes are called 'blips' and mean that you should have your viral load retested as soon as possible. Blips are often due to a problem with the testing equipment, but could be a warning sign of other problems, such as treatment failure, drug interactions, poor adherence or illness.

If you have two viral load tests at least a month apart and both show that your viral load is above 400, then a treatment change should be considered. It's recommended that you have a resistance test to see which of your drugs isn't working and to help you choose replacement drugs. These tests are only accurate if your viral load is above 1,000, and if you change drugs due to treatment failure without having a resistance test, it's recommended that your new treatment regimen consists of a completely new set of drugs.

If you have to change treatments because of side-effects and have an undetectable viral load, then it's completely safe to only switch the drug or drugs causing the problem.

Anti-HIV drugs have to be taken very consistently to work properly (this is called adherence), so if you haven't been taking your treatment properly for any reason, make sure that you switch to a new combination which is easier to take, and fits in with the way you live your life.

Changing treatment due to side-effects

Side-effects are the main reason why people change drugs in their first anti-HIV combination.

Although you may have a good viral load response after starting antiretroviral therapy, you may find the side effects of some drugs hard to live with. Changing treatment is an option if side effects cannot be controlled. If you viral load is undetectable the only drug you will need to change is the one causing the side-effects.

The main problem with changing treatment due to side effects is that the new combination may not be able to control HIV as well as the old combination. It is also possible that the new drug or drugs you switch to will bring their own unwanted effects.

There is also a bigger risk that the new combination will fail if you have lots of previous experience of treatment.

Switching from a protease inhibitor to a combination that doesn't include this class of drugs may bring about improvements in levels of fats in the blood (lipids). For more information see 'Changing treatment because of lipodystrophy'.

Changing treatment due to lipodystrophy

Lipodystrophy is the name given to a syndrome of side-effects caused by anti-HIV drugs. It includes an increase in fats in the blood (which can increase your long-term risk of a heart attack, diabetes and stroke), and changes in body shape (including fat loss from the face, limbs and buttocks), and fat gain (at the back of the neck - sometimes called buffalo hump - and around the stomach).

The NRTI d4T has been particularly associated with fat loss, and if you are taking d4T you are recommended to switch it for another drug, if you have treatment options available.

If you have high blood fats and are taking a protease inhibitor, then it might be worth switching to an NNRTI, if this option is available to you. Changes in your diet can also help, see the chapter *Nutrition and HIV*. Exercise can also be helpful and is looked at in more detail in the chapter *Exercise*. Your doctor can also prescribe drugs (called statins and fibrates) to control fats in your blood.

AZT has also been associated with fat loss, but at a slower rate, and if you are taking AZT you should have the risks of fat loss explained to you and given the option of switching to another drug.

Changing your treatment appears to have only a very minimal impact on body fat changes. Lost fat has been shown to slowly return to the limbs for two years after switching from d4T or AZT to abacavir or tenofovir. Fat loss can be very distressing, particularly fat loss from the face. The use of a cosmetic treatment called *New Fill* (polylactic acid) can help fill out the checks and remedy the wasted appearance that facial fat loss causes. Treatment involves a course of injections, and it may have to be repeated. Some, but not all, HIV clinics provide the treatment for free on the NHS, but some people have to obtain *New Fill* treatment privately. A single course of treatment costs from £800 - £1,200.

Surgery is sometimes used to remove fat which has accumulated around the back of the neck.

Fat loss and fat gain caused by anti-HIV drugs can be emotionally very distressing and uncomfortable. It's important that you let your doctor know how body fat changes are affecting you. If you have fat loss from the face or fat gain around the neck, your doctor may be able to refer you for cosmetic surgery to help correct it. Staff at hospitals with large HIV clinics are becoming very skilled at providing cosmetic treatments for fat loss and fat gain caused by anti-HIV drugs. Also make sure that you tell your doctor if changes in your body shape are causing emotional or psychological problems, as mental health support will be available.

Salvage therapy

If you are resistant to many anti-HIV drugs from more than one drug class, then you might find it harder to assemble a drug regimen which will get your viral load down to undetectable levels.

But it's still worth taking anti-HIV treatment. Even if your treatments are unable to achieve an undetectable viral load, your health is still likely to benefit. If you have limited treatment options, your CD4 cell count might be a better tool to assess the effectiveness of your treatment. Finding a new treatment regimen that will increase your CD4 cell count, your health, and your quality of life is likely to be a better option than trying to assemble a combination to control your viral load.

If you are resistant to drugs from all three main classes of anti-HIV drugs (NRTIs, NNRTIs and protease inhibitors), doctors often say you need 'salvage therapy'.

The more new drugs you can add to a combination, the more likely it is that your salvage regimen will work. Resistance tests should be used to help determine which drugs will work best for you. Tests to measure the amount of anti-HIV drugs in your blood may also be useful to ensure that you are taking the most effective dose of your medication.

If your HIV is resistant to a number of anti-HIV drugs, you may find it difficult to assemble a new regimen which can lower your viral load to undetectable levels. The aim of treatment should be to maintain or increase your CD4 cell count and to prevent you from becoming ill. Many doctors now also think that, newer drugs mean that it is possible to suppress viral load to undetectable levels and keep it there even in people who have taken many anti-HIV drugs before.

Structured treatment interruptions are not recommended if you are taking 'salvage therapy'.

If you are not at risk of rapidly becoming seriously ill because of HIV (for example you have a CD4 cell count above 100 which is not falling quickly) then you may wish to consider waiting until enough new drugs are available to give you a chance of getting your viral load below 50 for a sustained period before you start taking a new combination of drugs. Some people in this situation have been put on 3TC (lamivudine, *Epivir*) as a single drug. This is because resistance to 3TC seems to stop more extensive drug resistance developing. Doctors should not add a single drug which works into your combination to get a short-term reduction in your viral load.

Use of T-20 and tipranavir or TMC114

T-20 (enfuvirtide, *Fuzeon*) belongs to a new class of anti-HIV drugs called fusion inhibitors, and has been licensed for use in people who have very few treatment options. Unlike all the other anti-HIV drugs, T-20 needs to be injected, twice daily under the skin.

Trials have shown that the protease inhibitor tipranavir (*Aptivus*) combined with T-20, and other drugs which a resistance test has shown still work,

104

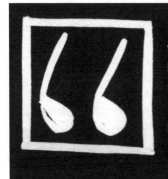

It is so hard, so very, very hard ... I worry all the time about my children back home. I really want to go, but I know if I did I would not live long. Staying here is the only way I can still be of help to my children.

positive voice

achieves the best results. Very good results have also been seen when T-20 is used with the as yet unlicensed protease inhibitor, TMC114 (*darunavir*).

If you are taking T-20 and it is the only anti-HIV drug that you are sensitive to, then you'll rapidly develop resistance to it. But even in these circumstances if you have a very low CD4 cell count and no other treatment options, it might prove to have some benefit.

Treatment breaks

There's been a lot of discussion about the value and safety of taking a supervised break from your HIV treatments (called a structured treatment interruption). The consensus now is that they may have more risks than benefits.

Doctors had hoped that taking structured treatment breaks would help to prime the immune system to control HIV without the use of anti-HIV drugs. Studies have shown that this is not the case.

However, another reason why some people are interested in them is the opportunity they may give individuals to take a break from anti-HIV treatment and its side-effects.

The potential benefits of a structured treatment interruptions were thought to be a boosted immune system and fewer side-effects.

Structured treatment breaks also have risks. Some people have reported complications, including a rapid fall in their CD4 cell count, illness due to HIV and the development of more drug resistance.

Recently a big international trial called the SMART study, which used CD4 cell counts as a guide to stopping and restarting HIV treatment, was stopped early when it was found that people taking a break from treatment were much more likely to become ill not only because of HIV but due to other serious causes as well. Another treatment interruption study conducted in Africa - an arm of the DART study - was stopped soon after when it was shown that people who took treatment breaks after fixed cycles of treatment were more likely to develop AIDS-defining illnesses.

If you are considering taking a break from your treatment, make sure that you discuss it carefully with your doctor beforehand.

Don't take a break from your treatment if your CD4 cell count is below 200 - there's a very real risk that you could develop a very serious infection. Treatment breaks are not recommended for people who need 'salvage therapy'.

If your lowest ever CD4 cell count was below 200 you are at higher risk of developing AIDS-defining illnesses during a treatment break.

Further reading

- NAM factsheets, *Anti-HIV therapy, Changing treatment* and *Treatment interruption.*

- *Anti-HIV drugs, Clinical trials, HIV therapy* and *Lipodystrophy,* booklets in the information for HIV-positive people series produced by NAM.

- 'Anti-HIV therapy' in NAM's *HIV and AIDS Treatments Directory.*

  African men and combination therapy, African women and combination therapy, Gay men and combination therapy, Starting, Changing, and *Sticking with it,* booklets produced by the Terrence Higgins Trust.

First refusal
by Alan

I first refused any HIV drug therapy. The only treatment available was AZT in strong doses and from all that I'd read, although it might have delayed AIDS a bit, it was at the price of toxicity. So while my CD4-cell count remained reasonably high, I wasn't going to start any therapy. The important thing was regular monitoring every six months. I also kidded myself that I was going to be the exception and that my immune system would be strong enough not to absolutely succumb to the virus.

It was a numbers game. CD4-cell scores fluctuated between 450 and 800 and viral load between 2000 and 20,000. When it did hit 20,000 after eight years my consultant at the time was very keen that I get onto treatment. No way, I told myself, not without another viral load test. To my relief, it dropped back down. However, when the CD4-cells dropped below 250 and my viral load was hitting over 100k the alarm bells were clanging. I'd managed thirteen years without treatment.

Once you start that's it, treatment for life. Then there is the side-effects issue and whether you're going to be able to keep up the discipline. It meant facing up again to the reality that I really was ill and that the condition would get me if I didn't act. The only way was to have a positive approach. Actually I had three key positives. These were the confidence I had in my then consultant; the support of my partner (now civil partner); and my ability to stick to something once I started it. The hospital put no pressure on me about starting HIV treatment. Their advice was that it was time to start treatment, but it was my decision. The pharmacists at the hospital were also unbelievably careful and caring; talking to me about my drug regime and how best to make sure I kept to routine. They answered question after question.

I'd had many healthy, treatment free years. If I now started HIV treatment, there seemed to be no reason why I shouldn't stay well and live a normal life. It seems like an easy decision, but it still felt momentous.

The side-effects of nausea and some diarrhoea went on for about three weeks. The nausea was particularly awful. I just mentally gritted my teeth and tried to carry on with whatever I was doing knowing that the waves of nausea would pass after many minutes and that it was worth persevering with the drugs for the long term health. The tablets, fortunately only two twice a day, have become just part of the daily routine like breakfast or watching the news.

Starting treatment
by Christopher

Following my HIV diagnosis in August 2001, my doctor estimated that I would be looking to start therapy in around six years. But following a rapid CD4 cell decline, it was only nine months later that he suggested I start thinking about choosing a drug regimen.

It's an understatement to say that I was disappointed with the way things had gone. I'd spent the previous year or so trying to find out as much as I could about HIV and its treatment - as a pharmacologist working in a university laboratory I felt at home with the scientific and clinical literature and was encouraged by what I had seen.

But when the imminence of my own HAART debut was staring me in the face, my level-headedness flew out of the window. It was like a second diagnosis. I was really scared.

For the next year or so, I regularly visited a treatments adviser at the clinic. She talked me through the various drug options available to me, and we eventually decided on a regimen of efavirenz and *Combivir*. While I was aware of the potential neuropsychiatric side-effects of efavirenz, protease inhibitors - particularly the threat of lipodystrophy - terrified me.

The year or so of two-monthly visits to the clinic were an exercise in procrastination. Every time I went back, I produced another excuse for delaying therapy - while they seemed genuine reasons to me at the time, it's clear to me now that I was avoiding facing up to my predicament. So, while my CD4 count hovered around the 200 mark, my adviser's patience eventually began to wear thin. Eventually my excuses ran out and, armed with a carrier bag full of pills, I reluctantly fixed a date to start.

I took my first *Combivir* pill during a coffee break at work. I spent the next four hours gazing out of my office window, waiting for the nausea to kick in, or to be rushing to the toilet with diarrhoea. They never came.

In the evening, I swallowed my first dose of efavirenz along with my second *Combivir* pill, half-expecting hellish nightmares and night sweats or suicidal feelings in the morning. After sleeping like a baby, I spent the next day feeling a little like I had smoked a joint in the morning - precisely as my adviser had warned me I would. The feeling was far from unpleasant.

The stoned feeling had worn off by the end of the day, and the morning grogginess disappeared entirely within three days. I tentatively started drinking alcohol again a few days later, with no unexpected effects, and rekindled my nocturnal dancing habits within two weeks - to find that "the efavirenz feeling", rather than forcing me to curtail my nights out, had added an interesting twist to the 4am taxi ride home.

I've now been on my combination for 18 months. It reduced my viral load to undetectable levels immediately, although its effects on my CD4 count took almost a year to kick in. Now, my CD4 count is marching up at a respectable pace, and I'm still free of side-effects.

Sure, I sometimes have diarrhoea, and I've had a bout of distressing nightmares recently. It's all too easy to put these down to the drugs and feel sorry for myself. But I try to remember that I've always had diarrhoea occasionally, and I remember worse dreams from my pre-HAART days.

My only regret is that I didn't start HAART little earlier, to increase my chances of a sustainable response to my current and future drug regimens - my CD4 count dipped below 200 on more occasions than I would like while I procrastinated. But at the time I didn't have the benefit of hindsight, so now the best I can do is enjoy these side-effect-free years, and hope that my next combinations will be as easy as my first.

Finally undetectable!
by Edwin

After almost 15 years of HIV, and six years of viral load testing, I heard on Thursday, June 21st 2001 that my viral load had dropped to an undetectable level for the first time. It was a milestone neither I nor my HIV consultant ever expected me to reach.

Fifteen months earlier I had taken a planned treatment interruption, and went off all antiretrovirals for a year. I had been on a variety of treatments, beginning with AZT monotherapy, since 1993. When the HAART era began, I had already become resistant to protease inhibitors, due to suboptimal early dosing of saquinavir, and by 1999 I was resistant to all three classes of currently available drugs. My liver also needed to recover from a (mitochondrially) toxic d4T/3TC combo.

Taking the treatment break wasn't an easy decision, but with my liver about to explode, apparently, and a rising viral load, there seemed to be little choice. I kept going with acupuncture and herbs, managed a once-in-a-lifetime Millennium trip to Australia, and then, once my viral load began to hit the half-million mark, slowly began to fade.

I used all of what little energy I had to read everything about the latest treatments, including everything from NAM, and reviewed all my resistance tests. In February 2000, *Kaletra* (lopinavir/ritonavir) became available in Canada (where I was living at the time) on expanded access. Together with my HIV consultant, we settled on restarting with five drugs, recycling several older options, and including a completely experimental drug called mycophenolate.

Amazingly, my liver didn't explode, and although I had the usual nausea and diarrhoea associated with starting a new regimen, within a few weeks I felt human again. After a month, my viral load plummeted from over 600,000 to the 5,000 range. My CD4s began to slowly increase, but I decided to try and throw everything at the virus in order to give me the best chance of a full immune recovery.

A few months later, during a holiday in Spain, I added another three drugs, making eight in total. I was nervous adding more away from home, but since I was British, I naively figured I could get free hospital treatment in Spain if there were problems. Fortunately there weren't, and, frustratingly, my viral load settled, remaining between 100-500 for the rest of 2000.

I was one of the first to be offered therapeutic drug level monitoring in early 2001, and we discovered that all my measurable drug levels were far too low, despite above-average doses of *Kaletra*. My viral load finally reached undetectable after further adjustments, and another day of therapeutic drug monitoring.

From being at death's door in March 2000, with a CD4 count of 30, I felt like I got my life back by the summer of 2001, with 210 CD4s. Most amazingly, my liver function tests were completely normal.

Therapeutic drug monitoring, along with Virtual Genotype testing, a great consultant, great GP, amazing partner and, above all, an almost pathological determination to beat HIV, got me to that point. Today my viral load is still undetectable and I'm taking "only" six different antiretrovirals and two lipid-lowering pills as well as testosterone injections in order to live a full and happy life!

If anyone tells you that all that is left is palliative care and you're not ready, or you are too frightened to try new treatments, don't give up. For me, at least, the fight was worth it.

Robert and treatment

I was diagnosed HIV-positive in 1997. I'm now 65. It was a bit of a shock. It could never happen to me, after all. I only found out because of someone's kindness and honesty.

In the autumn of 1997, I had felt really out-of-sorts; I developed a flu (which I'd never had before) and came out in a rash - which I now know was probably the HIV starting. I got over that, but still felt awful. The "someone" kept asking me to go over, as he wanted to tell me something "important", but I just didn't feel up to it.

Anyway, eventually I did go, and he said something like "I've something to tell you." He said that he had been diagnosed HIV-positive on his annual test. So I had "the test" too, and learned that I was HIV-positive.

My blood tests showed that my viral load was 500,000 and my CD4 cell count was 210! I was put on anti-HIV drugs immediately. The drugs were indinavir, AZT, and ddI. I hated the regime because of indinavir, and its eating restrictions. Anyway, I carried on enthusiastically with my job as a lecturer in computing subjects at a local college of further education.

Side-effects developed, though my viral load came down to 'undetectable' in six months and my CD4 count went up to

400. I became very weak in my legs - I could hardly climb onto a stool, or get up if I was lying sunbathing! Also, my cholesterol level went up sharply, which was actually the saving of me!

The clinic altered my treatment because of the rise in my cholesterol levels, replacing the indinavir with efavirenz.

What a relief! No restrictions, and all my strength came back. I don't 'work out', but always do sensible things like cycling a bit, walking, eating well (and enjoying wine and beer). I don't take drugs or smoke.

Eventually, a job was advertised for a network manager for a nearby comprehensive school, and, again being very positive in my life attitude, I applied, and was accepted. I didn't disclose my HIV status, only my GP knows it. At first just me, my team has grown, and I love it!! I've been doing the job for over five years now.

I am a very happy sort of person, and hardly think of my HIV status. I just take the tablets (never missing a dose) and get on with my life. My viral load is still undetectable.

As Woody Allen said, "It's not that I'm afraid to die, I just don't want to be there when it happens".

From devastation to optimism

An HIV diagnosis is still a devastating experience and in the time before antiretroviral therapy it seemed like a death sentence. I was diagnosed in 1993 and informed my CD4 count was 9 and told I had two years at the most to enjoy what was left of my life. Before my diagnosis I felt I had the world at my feet and my life was blessed. As a consequence of this diagnosis I lost my health, career, relationship and home within a matter of months. Added to this I was caring for several friends in the advanced stages of AIDS, all of who subsequently died. I became acquainted with many churches and crematoria in the Greater London area.

I started taking *Septrin* as a prophylaxis against PCP and my system reacted badly. I had my first admission to an AIDS ward at St Marys hospital in Paddington in June 1994 and since then have been an in-patient more than thirty times, four of which I did not expect to survive. On many occasions I prepared for my death, planned my funeral and informed loved ones only to recover unexpectedly. I was becoming the boy who cried wolf.

Throughout all this I have had amazing support from family and friends which I feel has been the fundamental key to my survival. I looked so ill at times that there was no way I could keep it hidden. At first I found it difficult having to deal with their emotions but when they saw I didn't adopt a victim mentality they rallied to encourage and support me in any decisions I made about my treatment and care.

In 1999 I agreed to start antiretroviral therapy which at first I found difficult to adapt to but six years on I am still taking the same combination. In April 2002 I took a treatment holiday with the consent of my doctor but after two months I began developing skin problems and digestive issues.

My health is currently good and I am rebuilding my life. I have three voluntary jobs, a beautiful garden and am doing an NVQ computer course. I think less of dying and am coming to terms with the fact I may have a future. My HIV has not gone away but with continued treatment and the support of a loving family and group of friends I have become optimistic and less fatalistic!

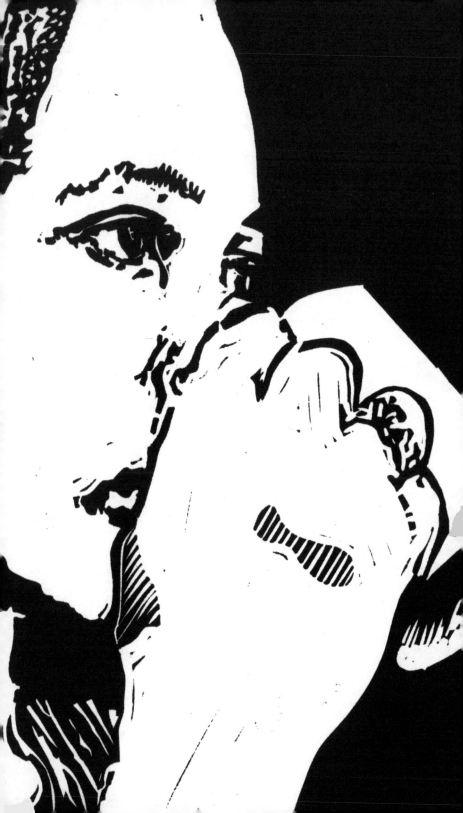

Adherence

taking your medicine

In this chapter you'll find information on

The importance of taking your anti-HIV
drugs properly to their effectiveness.

The minimum number of doses of anti-HIV
treatment you need to take.

Some things which might help you take your
drugs properly.

Why taking doses of your medication can be
as bad as not taking them at all.

Support your clinic should offer you.

Some practical adherence tips.

There is a testimony from a man about his
attitude towards adherence.

Introduction

Taking your anti-HIV medication properly is the single most important thing you can do to ensure the success of your anti-HIV treatments.

Adherence to your anti-HIV treatments involves the following elements:

- Taking all the drugs that make up your anti-HIV treatment regimen.
- Taking the right number of pills.
- Taking your drugs the correct number of times each day.
- Taking your drugs at the right time - (taking your medicines too late, or too early can be as bad as not taking them at all).
- Taking your drugs with or without food according to instructions.
- Making sure that your drugs don't interact with other medicines prescribed to you, or bought over the counter. Herbal remedies and recreational drugs can also interact with anti-HIV medication.

Why adherence is important

Not taking your HIV medications properly can mean that they do not work effectively, leading to an increase in your viral load, a fall in your CD4 cell count and a greater risk of becoming ill and dying because of HIV.

The reason adherence is so important is because HIV can quickly become resistant to the drugs used to treat it. If the blood level of an anti-HIV drug drops too low, then it will be unable to stop HIV reproducing and this gives the virus an opportunity to develop resistance. The drug-resistant strains of the virus will become dominant.

This could mean that not only do you become resistant to the drugs you are currently taking, but also to drugs similar to these. For example, if you develop resistance to one NNRTI, you're likely to become resistant to all NNRTIs. This is called cross-resistance, and although the risk varies from drug to drug, cross-resistance can occur in all classes of drug used to treat HIV.

Adherence is so important that many doctors think it is better to stop treatment altogether rather than miss doses. However, this carries its own risks, and if you are finding it difficult to take your medication and think that you need a break from your treatment, discuss the pros and cons with your doctor.

Level of adherence to aim for

You should try and take all your doses correctly. The best response to anti-HIV therapy is seen in people who had 100% adherence to their treatment. Levels of adherence of less than 95% have been associated with poor suppression of HIV viral load, rebound in viral load, and either poor CD4 cell gains or falls in CD4 cell count.

If you are taking your treatment once a day, 95% adherence means missing, or incorrectly taking, only one dose a month.

If you are taking your treatment twice a day, 95% adherence means missing, or incorrectly taking, only three doses a month.

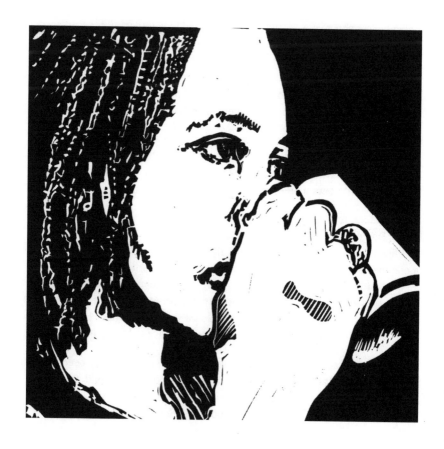

If you are taking your medication three times a day, 95% adherence means missing, or incorrectly taking, only four doses a month.

Adherence at this level can be very hard, and is much higher than the level needed for other medication. Nevertheless, try to take all your doses. Remember, any fall in the level of drug levels in your blood will give an opportunity for strains of HIV to develop which drugs don't work against.

How to boost your chances of adherence
You are more likely to adhere to your HIV treatments if you were involved in the decisions about both when to start treatment and about which drugs to start treatment with.

Being honest about your lifestyle to yourself and to your doctor can help ensure that you start on a combination that is right for you. Don't make unrealistic demands on yourself, and think about how taking medication will fit in with your social, working, eating and sleeping patterns. The chances are that there will be a combination available that will mean that you don't have to change your lifestyle at all, or make only modest alterations to your routine.

Side-effects are a very common reason why people skip doses. If you are experiencing side-effects of any kind, make sure you tell your doctor. The chances are that there will be another treatment option available. It's better to change treatments than miss doses and risk resistance.

Taking handfuls of pills is often cited by people as a reason why they miss doses. Doctors call the number of pills you have to take your 'pill burden'. If you find taking lots of pills a problem, then talk to your doctor about taking a combination with as few pills as possible. It might be that you can switch to a combination that involves taking no more than a couple of pills twice a day and by late 2006, potent HIV treatment that consists of just one pill, once a day is expected to be available. But make sure that you consider how these 'easy to take' regimens fit in with the reality of your day-to-day life.

Depression and other emotional and mental health problems have been linked with low levels of adherence. If you're depressed and don't think that you can cope with starting HIV treatments, then it might be best to wait until you feel more able to cope. Similarly, if you become depressed whilst taking treatments, it's important to seek help. Depression is very common in people with HIV (see the chapter on *Mental health*), and many HIV clinics have specialist mental health teams who can offer treatment and support. Treatments for depression work just as well in HIV-positive people.

Having problems with money and housing, and feeling isolated, have also been known to be associated with low levels of adherence in some people. Many HIV organisations can provide advice about money and accommodation, and your HIV clinic may even have a specialist HIV social worker you can see for advice. If you have family or friends who know that you are taking HIV-medication, try and talk to them about the problems you are experiencing - you might find that they are able to offer wonderful support. On the other hand, if you are worried about people close to you knowing that you have HIV, you might find that one solution is an adherence support group involving other HIV-positive people. These are organised by many HIV clinics and HIV support agencies.

Late doses

Taking your medication too late (or too early) can be as bad as not taking it at all, and can allow HIV to become resistant to some or all of the drugs you are taking.

The safest approach is to aim to take all your medicines at the right time and in the right way. But, being honest, there are bound to be times when you take your medicine late. As long as this happens very occasionally, it shouldn't make any difference to the success of your treatments. However, regularly taking your medication too late or too early will give HIV an opportunity to become resistant.

Not all anti-HIV drugs are processed by the body at the same rate. Protease inhibitors, especially those that aren't boosted by a small dose of ritonavir, are metabolised very rapidly, meaning that it's particularly important to take them correctly.

Other drugs, for example NNRTIs, are more forgiving and it's not quite so important to take them at very strict intervals - taking them an hour or so late shouldn't make too much of a difference.

> I have had no problems with my medications despite my dread of taking them. I know I'm lucky and it feels so unfair... They made my partner so sick all the time that he had no quality of life left. It broke my heart when he decided to stop taking them and I had to watch him die.
>
> positive voice

Don't assume that just because somebody else has taken their anti-HIV drugs constantly late and still has an undetectable viral load, that this will be the case for you, even if they are taking the same drugs as you. The speed and efficiency with which individuals process medicines can vary a lot.

If the way you live your life means that you find it very hard to stick to strict dosing schedules, then talk to your doctor about the possibility of switching to a more 'forgiving' combination.

Should you forget to take a dose of your drugs, take it as soon as you remember, and then carry on with your normal dosing schedule. Don't take a double dose to make up for the one you missed.

You might find that breaking your routine in some way increases the chances that you forget to take your pills on time. If you know that your normal dosing schedule is going to be disrupted, then try and make a plan that ensures you take your medication properly. If you do forget to take your dose, don't beat yourself up, but try and learn from it so it doesn't happen again.

Support from your clinic

If you understand why you are taking HIV treatment and why adherence is important, then you're more likely to take your treatments properly.

When you are first prescribed anti-HIV drugs, your doctor should explain when and how to take them. You should also be given written information to take away and read. This should help you to remember what the doctor told you.

You should also be told what side-effects to expect. Most HIV drugs cause unwanted side-effects, but on the whole these tend to be mild and go away over time. Knowing what to expect might make the side-effects easier to plan for and cope with. This should mean that you are more likely to think that they are worth getting through and so continue to take your medication.

In summary, when you first begin or, if you need to, change treatments you should understand:

- Why you have been given these drugs.

- How often you need to take them.

- If there are any dietary restrictions.

- If there are any side-effects and how to manage them (and when to seek urgent medical advice).

- Where you can get help and advice (including during normal working hours and at the evenings and weekends. Many hospitals have a 24-hour pharmacy support line).

Taking anti-HIV medication is likely to be a life-long commitment, and you may find that you need different levels of adherence support at different times. Make sure that you tell a doctor, nurse or pharmacist if you are having problems with adherence. They shouldn't judge you and will almost certainly be able to help.

Adherence tips

Simple forgetfulness is probably the most common reason why people miss doses of anti-HIV drugs. Don't give yourself too hard a time if this happens occasionally - you're only human, after all. But if it's happening often, talk to your doctor about it. It might be that you can change to a treatment combination that is easier to adhere to. If this isn't an option, then there might be some practical support that can be offered to help you manage your treatment better.

It could be that you just need a few prompts or reminders to boost your adherence. Listed below are a few strategies you might find useful.

Practice

Before you start taking a combination, if possible, practice for a few weeks before. For example, take sweets or multivitamins in the same quantities and at the same time as you would have to take your anti-HIV drugs. Make sure that you also follow any dietary restrictions.

Keep a diary

Have a written record of the doses you need to take. Tick off each dose as you take it. You can download a drug diary from the factsheets section at www.aidsmap.com.

Jog your memory

If you need a reminder, then setting an alarm on a watch might prove useful.

Pill boxes

You can get partitioned containers from your clinic to fill every week or few days with individual doses. Keep doses in different places where you might be when the time you need to take a dose comes around, for example at work, in your bag, or at a friend's house. Make sure that the container is suitable - pills can deteriorate if not stored properly - and remember that medicines have a use-by date. Make sure that you store medicines out of the reach of children, and avoid places that are very cold or hot.

Holidays, travel, and going out

Going away on holiday can have an effect on your adherence. Travelling long distances might disrupt your medicine schedule. Make sure that you take enough medicine with you, and always travel with your pills in your hand luggage. That way, it's closer to hand if you need to take it during your journey and is also less likely to get lost.

Holidays involve a break in routine, which could mean that you miss some of the prompts that remind you to take your drugs. It may help if you think in advance of other ways to remember them.

Taking your medicine away from home may mean that you will have to take it around people who don't know about your health, or whom you don't want to know. Plan in advance how to manage this. Simple things like having a bottle of water by your bed, and a handy snack like a chocolate bar, might give you the privacy you need to take your medicines.

Even going out for the evening can increase the chances that you might miss a dose. So make sure that you have any necessary medicine on you before you leave home. If you're going to a club and are likely to be searched, there's a chance that door staff might not recognise prescription medicines. There have been cases of people having their HIV medication confiscated by bouncers when trying to get into clubs.

Simply having a good time, particularly if you've been drinking or taking drugs, can also increase your chances of missing a dose. Try and have a prompt to remind you to take your medicines. Also remember that anti-HIV drugs and recreational drugs can interact. Ask your doctor or other member of your healthcare team if this is a concern for you. They should be able to offer advice about minimising the risk. Don't skip doses.

Further reading

- NAM factsheets, *Adherence, Adherence tips, Drug diary, Drug check-list* and *Late doses*
- *Adherence*, booklet produced by NAM.
- 'Anti-HIV therapy' in NAM's *HIV and AIDS Treatments Directory.*
- *Things to help you stick with it,* leaflet produced by the Terrence Higgins Trust.

Jewelled friends
by Alan

I have a pretty little carved wooden pill box which I'd bought in Eureka California. It holds my tablet set for the evening if I'm going out. My mobile phone is set to ring twelve hours apart to remind me; and my man reminds me too. A little obsessively, I snap the tablets from each blister sheet in an even order so I am confident I've taken one of each without having to count. Once I dropped one in the bedroom and wasn't happy until I found it in order to keep the sets even! I regard them as little white jewels to be treasured and respected. When I have a month's supply left I get slightly panicky and make sure I get another three months supply. When the box arrives by post it feels like receiving a present. They really are a gift. I feel very lucky I live in a country where I can get HIV treatment. The tablets look after me and keep me well - in fact I think of them as dear friends.

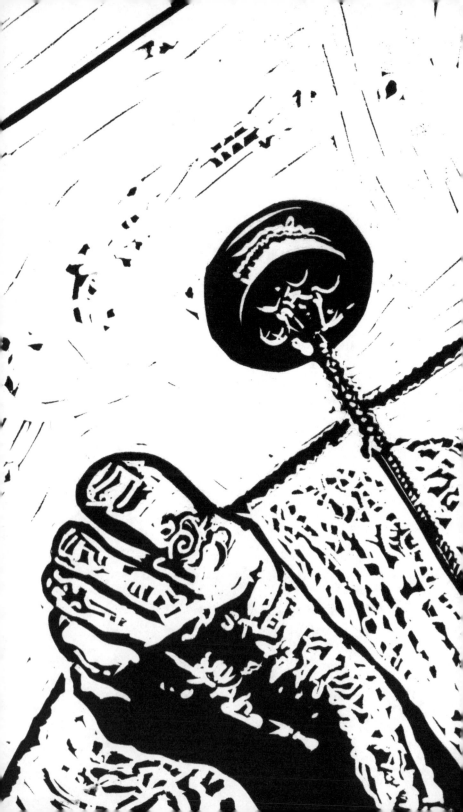

Side-effects

In this chapter you'll find information on

The types of side-effects you might
experience when taking anti-HIV drugs.

When side-effects might develop.

Three major side-effects which can develop
in people taking HIV drugs called
lipodystrophy, peripheral neuropathy
and nausea.

Four men write about their experiences of
side-effects.

Introduction

Nearly every medicine can cause unwanted side-effects in some people.

Side-effects are a common cause of illness, discomfort and distress in people taking anti-HIV drugs - even in people who have an undetectable viral load and high CD4 cell count and don't have any symptoms of HIV infection.

However, it's not inevitable that you will experience side-effects from any of the medicines you are given to fight HIV or other infections. It's also worth remembering that a lot of side-effects are mild, can be controlled with other medicines, and lessen or even go away over time.

Types of side-effects

There are two main reasons for side-effects: an allergic reaction to the drug which causes side-effects, or side-effects caused by the direct effects of a medicine.

An allergic reaction will cause side-effects such as a rash or fever. You should contact your doctor immediately if you suspect that you have developed an allergic reaction to any medicine you are taking. An allergic (hypersensitivity) reaction to abacavir (*Ziagen*) can be potentially fatal. If you are taking abacavir you should read carefully the warning card that comes with boxes of the medicines and contact your doctor immediately if you experience any symptoms suggesting that you might be experiencing an allergic reaction to the drug.

If a side-effect is being caused by the unwanted effects of a drug itself, the nature of the side-effect might depend on which part of the body the drug is intended to treat, or the way in which the body processes the drug. For example, some drugs can damage the cells in bone marrow which are responsible for producing new blood cells, so this could mean that your body doesn't produce enough red or white blood cells. Some medicines can make you feel generally unwell, or cause vomiting, nausea, or diarrhoea. Reduced sex drive or sexual problems are another common side-effect.

Side-effects are often related to the amount of drug you are taking - for some drugs, but not all, it is possible to adjust the dose you receive to help minimise the risk of side-effects.

When side-effects develop

Side-effects soon after starting treatment

Most side-effects occur after you have been taking a medicine for a week or two. However, there is no strict pattern, and some people develop side-effects after taking their first dose of a drug. For others, side-effects don't develop for many months.

Side-effects occur in the first month or so of taking a drug not because you are being poisoned by the medicine, but because you have especially high concentrations of a drug in your blood in the weeks and months after you first start taking it. Over time, the peak drug levels in your blood go down, and side-effects tend to wear off. Because of this, it might be recommended in some cases that you gradually increase the dose you take of a drug over a few weeks.

Side-effects are often worse during the first month or so of taking a drug. Over time, they may lessen, modify, or go away altogether.

Daily pattern to side-effects

There can be a daily pattern to side-effects, linked to the time you take your medicines and also to the processing of the drug by your body. It might be possible to minimise the inconvenience that this causes by adjusting the time at which you take your medicines. For example, the NNRTI efavirenz (*Sustiva*) can cause dizziness and other psychological side-effects. Many people overcome these by taking their daily dose of the drug just before going to bed.

Medicines to control side-effects

Medicines are available to help control side-effects in both the short and the long term. These include anti-sickness and anti-diarrhoea drugs.

Longer-term side-effects

It's also known that some side-effects only develop in the longer term. For example, lipodystrophy, changes in body shape and blood fats, has been seen in people taking anti-HIV drugs for a number of months or years. A rare, but serious long-term side-effect is called lactic acidosis. There's a lot more information about lipodystrophy later in this chapter.

Side-effects and a weakened immune system

If you have a very weak immune system there's some evidence to suggest that you might be more vulnerable to side-effects, including painful nerve damage to the feet (peripheral neuropathy) and fat loss from the face, when you start taking anti-HIV drugs if your immune system is already severely damaged by HIV. There's a lot more information about peripheral neuropathy later in this chapter.

Coping with side-effects

The risk of side-effects might be something you consider when deciding whether or not to take a certain treatment. If you are ill, or at risk of becoming ill, the benefits of the treatment may well be clear-cut and far outweigh the risk of side-effects.

If you have decided it is worthwhile taking a treatment and you do develop side-effects, it's important to establish which drug is causing the problem. This can be quite tricky if you are taking anti-HIV medication, as more than one of the drugs might have the potential to cause the side-effects you are experiencing.

Talk about problems you are experiencing with side-effects with your doctor. Don't stop taking treatments without seeking medical advice.

Taking other medicines, such as anti-sickness or anti-nausea medication, can help control side-effects.

If it's known that a particular anti-HIV drug is causing side-effects, then there's a good chance, particularly if you've never taken anti-HIV drugs before, that you will be able to switch to a drug that doesn't cause the side-effects you are experiencing.

Nausea, lipodystrophy and peripheral neuropathy

Three common and distressing side-effects of anti-HIV treatment are nausea, lipodystrophy (changes in body shape and increased blood lipids) and peripheral neuropathy (painful damage to the nerves in the feet, lower legs and, sometimes, the hands). Detailed information on these side-effects is provided below.

Nausea and vomiting

Many anti-HIV drugs are associated with nausea. However, it is most commonly reported as a side-effect of AZT (zidovudine, *Retrovir*), d4T (stavudine, *Sustiva*), 3TC (lamivudine, *Epivir*), and abacavir (*Ziagen*) from the NRTI class. Protease inhibitors which commonly cause nausea include indinavir (*Crixivan*) and ritonavir (*Norvir*) and those containing a small dose of ritonavir to boost their effectiveness. Some of the drugs used to treat infections commonly seen in people with HIV also cause nausea, including cidofovir, foscarnet, ganciclovir, intravenous pentamidine, co-trimoxazole and clarithronycin.

If nausea is accompanied by other symptoms, the underlying cause needs to be investigated and treated. If it is due to drug side-effects, then the dose and frequency may need to be altered or the drug discontinued. Don't alter the dosing of your treatments without discussing it with your doctor first.

Some drugs, e.g. AZT, can be taken with food in order to limit nausea. Talk to your HIV pharmacist or doctor about this to clarify which foods can be eaten with your medication, and which to avoid, or see *Nutrition* in NAM's information series for people with HIV.

Anti-nausea medication

Anti-nausea medication (sometimes called anti-emetics), taken either as tablets or injections, can be prescribed by your doctor to help manage symptoms. This can be particularly important when starting a new treatment, such as anti-HIV combination therapy, which is associated with a high risk of nausea and vomiting during the first few weeks. Adequate anti-nausea medication can help you adjust to your new regimen and make this initial period easier.

Many different drugs are used to treat nausea and/or vomiting. These include metoclopramide, prochlorperazine, perphenazine, trifluoperazine, chlorpromazine, domperidone, granisetron, ondansetron, tropisetron and nabilone.

Coping with nausea and vomiting

For some people, having to swallow large tablets or large numbers of tablets can itself bring on bouts of nausea. If you think this might be a problem for you, it might influence your choice of anti-HIV therapy. For example, you could ask to see the different drugs available and find out about the number of doses required.

Whatever the cause, do not feel obliged to "grin and bear it" - nausea and vomiting can prevent you from getting enough food and nutrients and from sticking with your chosen treatment regimen. As well as asking your doctor about anti-emetic medication, the following practical tips may be helpful and can be discussed with an HIV dietitian:

- Eat small, frequent meals throughout the day rather than two or three large meals.
- Don't eat liquid and solid food at the same meal. Space them at least one hour apart.
- Avoid eating greasy, fatty, fried or spicy food. Instead, choose bland food.
- Try dry food such as toast, crackers, cereal, and fruit and vegetables that are bland or soft.
- Salty food such as crackers, pretzels and popcorn can help reduce nausea. Carry a packet with you when you leave the house.
- Don't lie flat for at least an hour after you eat.
- Eat food cold or at room temperature - hot food can worsen nausea.
- Herbal tea (e.g. peppermint or chamomile) or root ginger can help settle upset stomachs.

Lipodystrophy

Changes in body shape and the metabolism caused by anti-HIV drugs are known as lipodystrophy. Only a minority of people who take anti-HIV drugs develop lipodystrophy.

Changes in body shape

Three different patterns of body fat change have been seen in people taking anti-HIV drugs. These are:

- Fat gain on the abdomen/belly, between the shoulder blades, around the neck, or in the breasts.
- Fat loss from under the skin which is most noticeable in the arms and legs, buttocks, and face, causing prominent veins in the limbs, shrunken buttocks, and facial wasting.
- A mixture of both fat gain and fat loss.

The fat gain in the belly which some people develop isn't made up of fat under the skin. Rather, it is caused by the build-up of fat within the abdomen. This makes the belly feel harder.

The majority of people who develop these changes experience a combination of both fat loss and fat gain, and you may often hear these body shape changes described as "fat redistribution".

A few people may also develop small, isolated fat deposits, called lipomas. Typically, these occur in the trunk and limbs.

Changes in body shape can be accompanied by changes in the body's metabolism.

The risk of developing body shape changes

It's not known exactly who will develop body shape changes whilst taking anti-HIV drugs. However, it seems that the risk is increased if you take a combination of anti-HIV drugs including protease inhibitors and NRTIs, especially d4T (stavudine, *Zerit*) or AZT (zidovudine, *Retrovir*).

It used to be thought that your chances of experiencing body fat changes were increased if you start taking anti-HIV drugs when you have a very low CD4 cell count. Recent research, however, suggest that it is drugs that are the cause of lipodystrophy.

It also seems that the following factors may increase your risk of body fat changes developing:

- Studies have shown that the longer you take anti-HIV drugs, the greater your risk of body fat changes occurring. One study showed that after three years of taking a combination which included a protease inhibitor and NRTIs, between 30%-40% of people developed some kind of body fat change. It's not known if the risk carries on growing after this point or if people who are likely to develop lipodystrophy will have done so by this point.

- People who are overweight seem more likely to develop central fat accumulation.

- Fat loss is more commonly reported in women.

- Older people are more likely to report both fat gain and fat loss from the limbs, buttocks, and face. It may be that some of these changes are, in fact, natural changes which occur with ageing.

Avoiding body fat changes

Because the reasons for body fat changes in people taking anti-HIV drugs aren't properly understood, it's very hard to give clear advice about how to avoid them.

It used to be thought that the changes were only seen in people who took protease inhibitors, but in fact the changes are seen in people who have never taken this class of drug.

However, it is known that protease inhibitors can disturb the way the body handles fats and sugars.

There is evidence that people who take d4T and, to a lesser extent, AZT are at greater risk of fat loss. It is also clear that people who start treatment with a combination that contains an NNRTI rather than most protease inhibitors are less likely to experience an increase in their blood fats and sugars.

Although you can delay the chances of developing lipodystrophy by not starting anti-HIV treatments, you need to balance this against the very real risk that you will become ill if you do not start anti-HIV drugs when you need them. Also, remember that fat loss seems to be more common amongst people who start anti-HIV treatments when their CD4 cell count is below 200.

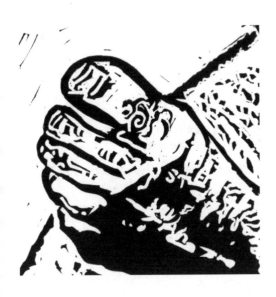

Changing treatment to avoid body fat changes

There's no really strong evidence to show that changes from a protease inhibitor to an NNRTI will lead to an improvement in body fat changes. There is, however, evidence that this strategy might lead to an improvement in blood fats and sugars.

Changing from d4T or AZT to abacavir (*Ziagen*) or tenofovir (*Viread*) can lead to a very slow recovery of fat loss.

Stopping treatment because of body fat changes

Because changes in body shape can be very distressing, some people choose to stop their anti-HIV treatment completely because of them.

There's no evidence that this will lead to an improvement in body shape changes, although it might help to normalise levels of blood fats and blood sugars.

If you are considering stopping treatment because of body shape changes, it is important that you are aware of the risks that this could involve and that you talk to your doctor about regular monitoring. If you stop treatment:

- Your CD4 cell count is likely to fall back to its pre-treatment level within six months or less, regardless of how high it is when you stop. It will continue to fall.

- If you had an AIDS-defining illness before you started anti-HIV treatment, you are five times more likely to experience a decline in your CD4 cell count to back below 200 (the point at which you become vulnerable to other AIDS-defining illnesses).

- If you stop treatment with a CD4 cell count below 200 then you are at risk of developing an AIDS-defining illness immediately.

- If you are taking drugs such as 3TC (lamivudine, *Epivir*), nevirapine (*Viramune*) or efavirenz (*Sustiva*), which take a long time to clear out of the body, you run the risk of developing resistance during the withdrawal period. If you want to start treatment again with the same drug or drugs, it or they may no longer work.

- If you start treatment again, your blood fats and sugars are likely to return to their normal level.

Treating fat gain

There are currently no treatments to reverse fat gain. Some people who stopped treatment completely have reported small improvements. Although changes in diet and exercise will help improve your overall health, they are not effective against fat gains caused by anti-HIV drugs.

There are, however, a number of experimental treatments which are being used to treat fat gain. These include human growth hormone, anabolic steroids, and a diabetes drug called metformin. Because these drugs haven't been proven to be effective against fat gain caused by anti-HIV drugs, you may only be able to get access to them if you enrol in a clinical trial designed to assess how good they are when used in such a way. Ask your doctor if this is possible.

Surgery is being as explored as a remedy for fat gain at the back of the neck.

Treating fat loss

Various treatments to restore fat loss is being examined.

In particular, several forms of facial reconstructive surgery have been used to help remedy the appearance of fat loss from the face. The most promising of these is called *New Fill* (polylactic acid).

Studies from the UK and abroad have shown that *New Fill* can reverse the appearance of facial wasting and lead to an improvement in a person's quality of life, self-esteem, and confidence.

New Fill is administered by a course of injections into the cheeks, normally spaced over several weeks. The injections fill out the sunken area and encourage tissue growth.

It's not known for how long treatment with *New Fill* will remain effective. So far, it seems that a single course of injections will help to remedy the appearance of fat loss from the face in most people for two years. However, it may last longer in some people. On the other hand, there have been reports of some people needing much more frequent treatment.

The most commonly reported side-effect is soreness and swelling in the area where the injections are given. *New Fill* is safe to use with anti-HIV drugs.

Access to *New Fill* from the NHS is limited. However, it's hoped that as more evidence about its effectiveness emerges, this will change. Some, but not all, HIV clinics will provide free treatment to their patients. If you cannot get it for free, private treatment costs between £800-£1,200 per course.

Other cosmetic treatments for facial wasting that are being considered include fat transfer, collagen injections and hyaluronic acid.

A dietary supplement called *NucloemaxX* is being explored as a possible treatment for fat loss from the limbs and buttocks. Some small studies have shown that the use of the supplement can lead to a modest improvement in fat in the arms and legs even when d4T and AZT are still being used.

Research suggests that a class of drugs called statins which are normally used to treat high levels of fat in the blood can also lead to a small improvement in fat loss caused by anti-HIV drugs.

Living with body shape changes

Body shape changes, in themselves, do not appear to be medically dangerous. However, they can cause physical discomfort and emotional problems. If you are becoming depressed because of changes in your body shape, make sure that you tell your doctor. Treatments for depression work well in people with HIV, and you might find a referral to see a counsellor or psychologist useful.

Changes in your metabolism

Anti-HIV drugs can also disrupt your metabolism - the way your body processes the things it needs to work properly.

Specifically, anti-HIV drugs can cause abnormal levels of blood lipids - cholesterol and triglycerides.

Cholesterol

There are two types of cholesterol. HDL cholesterol, often called good cholesterol, and LDL, or bad, cholesterol.

Levels of HDL cholesterol are often reduced in people with HIV and other chronic illnesses. High levels of LDL cholesterol indicate that you are at risk of heart disease, and increases of LDL cholesterol are often seen in people taking anti-HIV drugs.

If you have high LDL cholesterol, the following factors increase your risk of heart disease even further:

- Smoking.
- High blood pressure.
- A family history of heart disease.
- Being physically unfit.
- Age over 45 for men and age over 55 for women.
- Diabetes or insulin resistance.
- High blood sugars.
- Being very overweight, particularly with a lot of fat around the middle.
- Use of stimulant recreational drugs like cocaine or amphetamines.

It is particularly important to monitor LDL cholesterol levels if you are taking a protease inhibitor.

Triglycerides
Triglycerides are fatty acids derived from fat, sugar and starches in food. These travel through the bloodstream and are stored in tissues or in the liver.

Glucose
Glucose is a form of sugar found in the blood. High levels of glucose can increase the risk of heart disease.

Insulin
Insulin is the substance produced by the body to control glucose levels in the blood. Some people taking anti-HIV drugs need to produce more insulin to keep their blood levels of glucose normal. This is called insulin resistance. It may be necessary to have your insulin levels tested.

Symptoms of metabolic changes
Abnormal levels of fats and sugars in the blood can sometimes cause symptoms including:

- Tiredness.
- Dizziness (due to high blood pressure).
- Loss of concentration.
- More frequent urination.
- Thirst.

However, some people don't notice any symptoms, even when they've had abnormal levels of fats and sugars for a long time and are at risk of heart disease.

Heart disease and anti-HIV drugs

Levels of fats in your blood may start to rise when you start anti-HIV treatment, particularly if you are taking certain protease inhibitors. Sometimes they can increase so much that it's necessary to change your diet, start exercising, or take a medication to control them.

Large studies of people taking protease inhibitors have shown that they have a slight, but nevertheless significant, increase in their risk of heart disease.

If you have any existing risk factors for heart disease, your anti-HIV treatment should be carefully chosen to ensure that it doesn't raise risk even further.

You should have your cholesterol, triglyceride and glucose levels monitored each time you have a routine clinic visit.

Looking after your heart

There is a lot you can do to help keep your blood lipids within safe limits. The information on diet, exercise, and stopping smoking in this book is a good place to start.

Lipid-lowering drugs

If you have high blood lipids, your doctor might prescribe lipid-lowering drugs. These are used to treat heart disease and hardening of the arteries. Three classes of drugs are available:

- Statins. This class of lipid-lowering drug has been used successfully in people with HIV. Statins are particularly effective at reducing levels of LDL cholesterol. Most statins can interact with protease inhibitors, but the drug pravastatin can be safely used with protease inhibitors. The main side-effect of statins is muscle weakness. Liver and kidney functions also need to be monitored.

- Fibrates. This class of drug lowers triglycerides and can also effectively lower LDL cholesterol. However, fibrates should not be taken if you have liver of kidney problems or if you are pregnant. On the other hand, fibrates seem less likely than statins to interact with protease inhibitors.

- Fish oil. A fish oil preparation that is rich in omega-3 fatty acids can reduce elevated triglycerides. However, you need to take a large number of pills every day for it to be effective. Fish oil can increase levels of HDL cholesterol.

Some drugs are also being investigated to see how effective they are at controlling glucose and insulin in HIV-positive people. These include metformin, sulphonylureas, and glitazones.

Peripheral neuropathy

Nerve damage can be a very painful side-effect of some anti-HIV drugs, and can also be directly caused by HIV itself.

Neuropathy is damage to the nerves. Nerves transmit signals within the brain and spinal cord (the central nervous system or CNS), and extend from the CNS to the muscles, skin and organs. The nerves that are outside the CNS are called the peripheral nervous system (PNS). They detect sensations, such as pain, and control movement.

Some of the peripheral nerves control body functions over which we have no conscious control, such as blood flow to the organs or the movement of food through the intestines. This is called the autonomic nervous system.

Symptoms

Peripheral neuropathy usually involves damage to the nerves in the feet or, less commonly, the hands. The symptoms can range from mild tingling and numbness through to excruciating pain that makes it impossible even to wear a pair of socks. Usually both sides of the body are equally affected.

Occasionally the autonomic nervous system can be affected, causing symptoms such as dizziness, diarrhoea and sexual dysfunction (inability to obtain or sustain an erection).

Neuropathy as a side-effect of anti-HIV drugs

Among people with HIV, neuropathy is commonly caused by certain medical treatments. It is a significant side-effect of several anti-HIV drugs - in particular, ddI (didanosine, *Videx*), d4T (stavudine, *Zerit*) and, to a lesser extent, 3TC (lamivudine, *Epivir*).

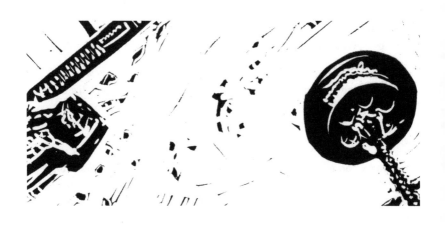

It can also be caused by other drugs prescribed for people with HIV, such as the antibiotics dapsone and intravenous pentamidine, the anti-TB drug isoniazid, and the anti-Kaposi's sarcoma drugs, vinblastine and vincristine.

If you take more than one of these drugs, the risk of developing neuropathy may be increased. If you have previously had neuropathy caused by something else, such as HIV itself, you may also be more likely to develop neuropathy from taking one or more of these drugs.

If you do develop drug-related neuropathy, it is important to stop taking the drug(s) promptly (but do try to get your doctor's advice before making any changes to your medical treatment). Once the drug has been stopped, the neuropathy may continue to get worse for a couple of weeks, but then it nearly always goes away over time. Later, you may be able to go back onto a reduced dose of the drug(s) without the neuropathy returning.

In the meantime, your doctor can prescribe treatments to reduce the pain, such as carbamazepine or amitriptyline. In severe cases, you may need strong painkillers. Trials have shown that a drug called *L-Acetyl-Carnitine* can help reduce the symptoms of neuropathy.

Other causes

There are several different causes of nerve damage among people with HIV.

Some causes are not linked to having HIV. For example, anyone who consumes large amounts of alcohol or certain recreational drugs like cocaine, heroin or speed can develop neuropathy; the best treatment is to stop or reduce your intake of these substances. Alcohol-induced neuropathy needs specific vitamin treatment from a doctor.

Neuropathy can also be caused by a shortage of vitamin B12, which can be relatively common among people with HIV. If medical tests confirm that you have a vitamin B12 deficiency, your doctor may offer supplements of vitamin B12 by injection (tablets are largely ineffective because vitamin B12 is poorly absorbed in the gut). Increasing the vitamin B12 content of your diet may also help a little; foods that are rich in the vitamin include fish, dairy products, kidneys, liver, eggs, beef and pork. Ask to see a dietitian at your clinic for more advice.

Some infections can cause neuropathy directly, such as cytomegalovirus (CMV) or HIV itself. These cases are best treated by tackling the underlying cause, such as using anti-CMV drugs or anti-HIV drugs, respectively

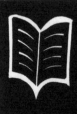

Further reading

- NAM factsheets, *Blood pressure, Blood problems, Cholesterol, Diarrhoea, Facial wasting, Fatigue, High blood pressure, Hyperbilirubinaemia, Lactic acidosis, Lipodystrophy, Nausea and vomiting, Neuropathy, Pain* and *Stroke.*

- *Anti-HIV drugs, HIV therapy,* and *Lipodystrophy,* booklets in the information for HIV-positive people series produced by NAM.

- 'Anti-HIV therapy' in NAM's *HIV and AIDS Treatments Directory.*

- *Why don't I feel better?,* leaflet produced by the Terrence Higgins Trust.

New life, *New Fill*
by Edwin

I had almost died in 2001, but thanks to an eight-drug salvage regimen I came back to life. Still my body and face bore the scars of lipodystrophy: thinning legs and bum, evidenced by varicose veins in my shins; central fat gain, evidenced by the increasingly larger jeans and baggier T-shirts I needed to hide my growing belly; and then, finally, deep lines in sunken cheeks and the shape of my skull obvious at my temples. I started seriously working out at the gym and changed my diet, gaining muscle where some of the fat used to be in my thighs, bum, and arms, and I soon lost much of my central fat accumulation. But my face remained lined and I felt that I had lost my looks - something that, as a vain gay man, bothered me more than I care to admit. And as an eight-year relationship came to end in the winter of 2001, I felt that I was now destined to live this hard-gained new life alone.

I found myself not being able to look at photographs of myself that showed me smiling, since the lines in my face deepened. In fact, as I stood in front the mirror pulling back the skin on my cheeks to see what my face had looked like before, I made a decision to try and smile less in general.

At first, I turned down an offer of *New Fill* from my Brighton HIV doc, saying that there must be much worse cases of facial wasting than mine. But after meeting an acquaintance who had had the treatment, and was glowing with confidence, I found the guts to ask for *New Fill* and in February 2003, I had my first appointment with Dr Gillian Dean - Brighton's *New Fill*-experienced doctor.

The treatment was not pain-free, but not as bad as root canal treatment at the dentist. But after the treatment was over, I was led into a small room and left alone with a mirror. It didn't really register at first that it was I who looked back at myself. Then I noticed how full my cheeks looked -almost too full, actually. Had I turned into a chipmunk? Was this Dr Dean's first disaster? I turned away and looked back again, this time more admiringly. Yes, the wasting was gone, but as Dr Dean explained when I subtly mentioned how full my cheeks looked, the effect at first is the bulk of liquid that contains *New Fill*. After a while, the liquid becomes absorbed and what is left is a thickening of the skin: that is why it takes three or four New Fill treatments to reach the required thickness.

That night, I looked at myself for a long time and realised that what the New Fill had done was not just fill my face and erase what I considered to be battle scars inappropriate to the way I wanted to live my life today, but also give me back the self-confidence that the lipodystrophy had imperceptibly eroded.

Chris's peripheral neuropathy

My peripheral neuropathy was caused by d4T, or was it ddI? I forget, it's such a long time ago.

The peripheral neuropathy I've experienced is different from that caused by HIV. The pain I've experienced sears through my big toes and top of my feet like hot cinders. It's transitory, passing in barely a second.

It doesn't sound like much, and goes unnoticed by people around me. Not surprising, as it normally just causes an involuntary twitch of the foot or leg.

My pain affects both big toes, and both feet, usually at the same time. It shoots across my instep and up into my calf muscles. There's no way of predicting when the pain will occur or how long it will last for.

The problem's not just the experience of the pain. It's what it does to me. It saps my will to live. I wilt, I lose my ability to concentrate, I'm overcome by a desire to collapse into sleep. This can last for a whole day - a whole day I'll never have again.

There are other physical symptoms as well. But these are more an expression of the emotional pain that peripheral neuropathy causes me. The pain forces a moan from my throat, my eyes smart with a deep searing wetness. Like the twitch in my leg or foot, all this goes unnoticed by the world around me.

People try to be helpful. A concerned friend recommended ibuprofen. "It's not that kind of pain", I reply. I don't think she understood.

Michael
what he did about his peripheral neuropathy

I took anti-HIV drugs in the belief that they would make me better. And true enough, within weeks of starting them my viral load fell back to undetectable and my CD4 cell count started a steady rise, banishing the minor illnesses which were plaguing my everyday life.

Well, something else started to plague my everyday life, and that was peripheral neuropathy. Quite simply it was the worst pain I've ever been in, and no painkiller, over-the-counter or prescription, seemed to make the slightest bit of difference.

To start with, I was reluctant to admit I had a problem. My test results were just so good. I didn't want to do anything which might give HIV a chance again. However, the pain became so bad that after a month of suffering I told my doctor how much pain I was in.

Without a moment's hesitation he recommended a treatment change. There were, he stressed, other drugs available, and there was no need to for me to suffer.

I still had my doubts. Both the drugs offered to me as alternatives - AZT and abacavir - seemed to have their own problems. However, my pain was such that eventually I opted for abacavir.

My viral load remained undetectable and my CD4 count continued to rise, and my peripheral neuropathy started to heal - very, very slowly. However, even though it's now years since I changed treatment I still have numbness and occasional pain in my feet. I've learnt that there's nothing to be gained from toughing through side-effects and that if you can do something about them, you should do it.

It's all arse over face
by Myles

"God, you look slim - you've lost so much weight!"

If I'd been overweight to start with, then that would fabulous. But you see, I'm over six foot tall and my weight started off at twelve stone. Reducing it to ten and a half could hardly be described as a good move.

You can never be too rich, too tanned or too slim, the saying goes. Rich, of course. Tanned , bring it on. But too thin, no.

Some drug company adverts make HIV treatment seem like a glamorous accessory. I'd would rather not have an accessory that gives me side-effects.

Seriously though, HIV treatment has given me the blessed opportunity in life to carry on and see my nephews grow, and maybe, let me have the opportunity to grow, very, very old.

It is finding the balance of how much long-term damage these little known about pills do, against the short to medium term benefits.

What is for certain, is that after almost eight years being diagnosed, I am still here and have avoided being "ill."

That sounds all good, but the journey of not getting "ill" to date has been patchy. Almost like finding your way across to a bit of London you are unfamiliar with. Car, bus, tube or train, which one to choose? Clearly you take the most comfortable and quickest. Discovering how is the hard work and takes time and patience.

In terms of HIV, this started in a car journey on very bald tyres that burst and crashed into a bout of peripheral neuropathy. I jumped on the tube and found a very cheery acupuncturist who after about a year got my feet back to some semblance of normality. That dull ache was pretty unpleasant and the ease that came with acupuncture was a welcome relief.

Next stop by plane to San Francisco. I was wide eyed and excited in 1999 to see bus shelters advertising HIV treatment. Young, tanned and toned sailors, pulling at the rigging on their round the world yacht race. HIV treatment was being glamourised, and desperately needed positive images of people with HIV were being provided.

And why not. Why should anyone be made to feel like a washed up pariah of society?

I came back to London with new information, always a stronger position to be in. My peripheral neuropathy had been "sorted," or was as good as it was going to get.

Everything I have read regarding HIV has always stressed the importance of strong working relationships with your consultant. I have been very lucky with my level of care. I know some are not as lucky. But come on, look at how poor access to HIV care is in Africa, China, Russia and India. How fortuitous are we to live in the UK?

Heads together, me and my consultant came up with a relatively easy triple combination. It steered away from protease inhibitors (which were then particularly associated with lipodystrophy - vanity is one of my characteristics). However, it did include AZT and that was to have consequences later.

In 2004, almost five years to the date that I travelled to San Francisco and saw the glamorous ads for HIV drugs and started my new combination. It worked - my viral load fell and my CD4 cell increased.

But on the down side, my triglycerides kept on increasing. Oh, and I had a very sore arse.The triglycerides were a worry, but I had to balance that against the success of the treatment. I was so sensitive about HIV making me ill that a mere spot would have me crawling the walls with worry.

And sitting at my desk for hours caused my bum to hurt. People would pass comment at how slim I looked, and I had spent time looking over my shoulder into the bathroom mirror, genuinely horrified at what I saw. My partner at the time made references to it and joked upon its appearance. I never found it funny.

My face was also changing. Small indentations were beginning to grow round the corners of my mouth - a cross between Robbie Williams and the joker from Batman. Now your arse you can cover, but not your face.

In fact, I felt pretty awful about it all. I could actually feel the cells in my glutes and down the backs of my legs being broken down. That "being eaten away" at feeling is repulsive. Like seeing maggots wriggle away at a piece of torn flesh from an animal carcass.

In seven years of being diagnosed, I had never "lost it".

Seeing your body change so much and conscious of the effects of medication, I finally, and thankfully, let the reservoir of professionalism, smiles that everything was okay, fear of not wanting family and friends to worry, break away.

In fact it didn't break, it exploded - the shit hit the fan.

A long story short, in quick succession I found myself off the pills and into a drug holiday. AZT had been found guilty of the crime of lipoatrophy - the medical name for fat loss - and was whisked off to drug heaven, or hell?

I would have preferred a holiday at the Hyatt, but hey, you've got to take what you can. The triglycerides came down very quickly, but I was left with a bizarre feeling of not having the crutch of pills, no longer being dominated by time, no more worries when I was away on business thinking what time I needed to take my pills in a different time zone. Yes, I hear you say, that's good. Good it is, yes, but very strange, almost like losing a bad mate; it left a big hole of nothingness.

During the summer I saw a professional counsellor, to help me understand how HIV and its enemy pills had consumed every square inch of my head. It needed to be compartmentalised into manageable, bite size chunks. My local HIV trust kindly organised this for me who were a great support.

I still, literally, have a pain in the ass, but at least I know it is not suffering any more damage.

The face is a bit different. I saw the look of shock on my mother's face back then, and knew what she was thinking.

I was paid a great compliment a month ago when she saw me and noted elatedly how I had "filled out". I knew I must have looked more like my old self. You don't realise the change so much when you see yourself every day. The gauntness had reduced. It's not how it used to be, but certainly not as bad as it was before I stopped my combination.

So much focus in the media is placed on the benefits of HIV treatment - and rightly so. But far less is placed on the how it can affect the way you feel about yourself.

Don't feel like you don't have an option. I didn't feel like I did, and it all ended in a mess of tears, runny noses, and feeling exhausted.

That's bullshit; life is too short. In this short life, everyone has the right to be confident in how they look, feel and portray themselves. Because if you don't, then that really is bullshit.

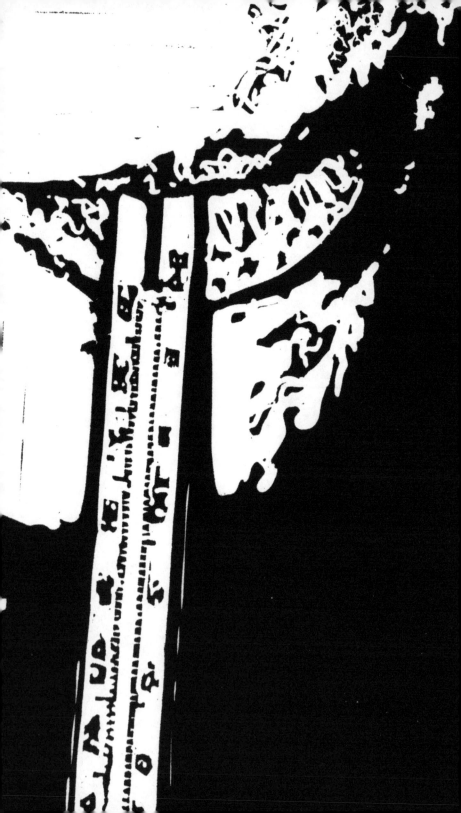

Symptoms and illnesses

In this chapter you'll find information on

Symptoms commonly seen in people
with HIV.

AIDS-defining illnesses.

Cancers seen in people with HIV.

Hepatitis coinfection in people with HIV.

Six HIV-positive people write about their
experiences of illness.

Symptoms

It's worth knowing the range of symptoms you might experience so that you can seek medical advice as soon as possible when you need it.

People with HIV get all the routine illnesses such as colds and flu that HIV-negative people get. So a chesty cough or diarrhoea could just be the result of the latest bug doing the rounds. But it could be something more serious, particularly if you have a low CD4 cell count. If your symptoms last for more than a few days, then you should see your doctor as quickly as possible.

What's more, anti-HIV drugs can cause side-effects. On the whole, these are minor and go away with time, but they can be more serious, and in certain circumstances dangerous.

Being able to get medical advice in an emergency is important. So it's worth finding out how you can get help from your clinic in an emergency or outside normal opening hours. You should also make sure that you are registered with a GP, who are the only doctors who can visit you in your home in the event of an emergency.

Doctors will always begin by asking you about your symptoms and examining you for signs of infection or allergy. They may then do a range of tests. Your doctor should explain what these tests are and why they are being undertaken.

Fevers and tiredness

These are sometimes called 'constitutional' symptoms because they affect the whole body. They can be the result of your body's attempt to fight an infection, and so can be caused by many different illnesses, and can also be caused by allergic reactions to some medicines.

Taking paracetamol can help reduce fevers, but should be used with caution by people with liver problems.

Night sweats

These are a common problem, and may be either mild and infrequent or quite severe, resulting in the need to change your bed linen or clothes.

Causes

If it is a new problem and accompanied by a fever, an acute infection is often the cause. More specific causes include tuberculosis and lymphoma. If the night sweats are intermittent and/or localised, then HIV infection is usually responsible; this is inconvenient but not a significant medical concern. Anxiety can also result in night sweats.

What to do

It is important to try to track down any infections (other than HIV itself) that could be causing the sweats, especially if they are accompanied by fever. Practical measures such as taking an aspirin or paracetamol before sleeping may be helpful. If the symptoms are severe and accompanied by other symptoms of HIV disease, then anti-HIV drug treatments may be considered.

Chest and breathing problems

Chest problems are very common and can be can caused by colds, flu, smoking, asthma, and bronchitis. However, people with HIV are particularly vulnerable to some potentially life-threatening chest infections, such as PCP pneumonia and tuberculosis. Coughs and difficulty breathing should be taken seriously, particularly if the symptoms last more than a few days. It's also worth knowing that breathing problems can be a symptom of a severe allergic reaction to certain medicines.

Standard tests used if you have chest or breathing problems include:

- Checking your temperature. A high temperature can be a sign that you have an infection, and if your temperature goes above 102, you should see your doctor as soon as possible.

- A blood count. A blood sample is taken to see if your red blood cells, which carry oxygen, are depleted.

- A chest x-ray. This will show if there is inflammation or fluid on the lungs.

- A sputum culture. A sample of spit or phlegm is taken to see if there is any sign of infection.

In some circumstances, you may need to have a bronchoscopy. This involves passing a very small tube down with a tiny camera attached down a nostril or the throat into the lungs. A small tissue sample, called a biopsy, may also be taken. Bronchoscopies are only performed if doctors are uncertain what the cause of a chest problem is. They can be uncomfortable and if you need to have one you will normally be offered *Valium*.

Skin problems
Skin problems are common in people with HIV.

A common skin complaint in people with HIV is seborrhoeic dermatitis. This can cause scaly patches on the skin, and can be successfully treated with ointments.

A red rash might be the result of an allergic reaction to a medicine. If this happens to you, see your doctor as soon as possible.

Small, painful blisters around the mouth, genitals and anus can be caused by herpes simplex virus. Herpes can be controlled using aciclovir (for more information see *Sex and HIV*).

Small colourless bumps on the skin with a pearly top can indicate that you have molluscum contagiosum (molluscum for short). You are particularly likely to get this if you have a low CD4 cell count, and they can spread around the body quite rapidly. They are treated by freezing them off or by surgery. If you develop them before starting anti-HIV treatment you may well find that they go away by themselves once your immune system strengthens.

Small cauliflower-like growths are probably warts. For more information see *Sex and HIV*.

Black, purple or dark brown spots on the skin can be a sign of the AIDS-defining cancer Kaposi's sarcoma (KS). To have this properly diagnosed, a sample of skin from the affected area needs to be biopsied. KS has become quite rare since effective anti-HIV treatments became available, but it can still be quite serious, so if you notice any unusual marks on your skin, make sure you bring them to your doctor's attention.

Mouth problems
Good dental hygiene including twice-daily brushing and flossing once a day will help you avoid most routine mouth problems.

However, people with HIV, particularly those with a low CD4 cell count, can be vulnerable to oral thrush, a fungal infection. Keep an eye out for white patches in the mouth. These can be painful, particularly if they are at the top of the throat, and can also cause an unpleasant taste. Oral thrush is easy to treat with a single dose of anti-fungal medication or lozenges. Once you start taking anti-HIV treatment and your immune system gets stronger, you'll probably find that you stop getting thrush.

If the white patches in your mouth are slightly hairy, then you might have an infection called oral hairy leukoplakia. This is caused by a virus and is treated with aciclovir. Again, you're likely to stop getting it once your immune system gets better after starting anti-HIV treatment.

Herpes blisters can affect the lips and mouth and can be treated with aciclovir. Mouth ulcers are more common in people with HIV, particularly people with lowish CD4 cell counts, but mouthwashes can help relieve the pain they cause. Mouth ulcers can also be a side-effect of some anti-HIV drugs.

Digestion problems
Pain or difficulty swallowing can be caused by oesophageal problems. The oesophagus is the tube that food passes down. Pain in the abdomen, nausea, vomiting, diarrhoea and constipation can all indicate stomach problems.

If these problems last more than a few days, or you start to lose weight, then see your doctor. Also, remember that most anti-HIV drugs can cause digestive problems, but these tend to pass with time and drugs can be taken to help control the symptoms.

Eye problems
You should have a periodic eye test, just like everybody else, to check your vision.

If you have a very low CD4 cell count, you should take problems with your vision very seriously. Blurred vision, blind spots, eye pain, or spots moving across the eye can all be symptoms of CMV (cytomegalovirus). This can be treated, but treatments work best if any eye damage is caught early.

Head problems
Everybody gets headaches from time to time. However, some anti-HIV drugs can cause problems with the head, as can certain infections, if you have a low CD4 cell count.

If you have any problems with your head lasting more than a few days, or any headaches which don't go away with normal painkillers such as paracetamol or ibuprofen, then see your doctor.

Side-effects caused by anti-HIV drugs tend to go away after time, and if they don't and you find that the head problems you are experiencing lower your quality of life, then speak to your doctor. It may be possible to change your medication.

Brain infections, such as toxoplasmosis and meningitis, are rare since the introduction of effective anti-HIV treatment. So too is AIDS-related dementia and lymphoma involving the brain. But if you experience symptoms of confusion, memory loss, poor concentration, speech problems or blackout tell your doctor immediately, particularly if you have a low CD4 cell count.

Depression is more common amongst people with HIV. For more information see *Mental health*.

Nerve problems
People with HIV can also experience problems with their peripheral nerves. This is called peripheral neuropathy, and it can be caused by HIV infection itself, or be a side-effect of drugs used to treat HIV and some other infections.

There is a lot more information on peripheral neuropathy earlier in this chapter.

Illnesses
The following is a summary of some of the more common illnesses that people with HIV can get. The list is not comprehensive, and it's worth remembering that the success of anti-HIV treatments means that many of the illness listed below are now very rarely seen in people with HIV in this country.

However, the PCP and tuberculosis both affect about 200 people a year in the UK. Cases of these illnesses often occur in people who are unaware that they are HIV-positive.

Treatments are constantly improving, so only very basic information about treatments has been included. More comprehensive information can be found on NAM's website www.aidsmap.com.

Most illnesses are caused by one of the following:

- A virus. These are simple organisms which reproduce using the building blocks of your own cells. This makes it very hard to get rid of them.
- Bacteria. These are single-cell organisms that antibiotics can kill.
- Protozoa and parasites. These are more complex organisms.
- Fungi. Yeasts and organic growths.
- Cancer. Cancers develop when your own cells develop out of control.

However, it's possible that you have already been infected with the organisms which cause many of the illnesses listed in this section. This is because they are very common across the population and only cause problems if the immune system is damaged and unable to keep them in control. Even then, there are sometimes effective treatments to stop the illnesses flaring up (preventative treatment or prophylaxis).

Candidiasis (thrush)
This is a fungus that can affect wet and warm surfaces, such as the mouth, throat, vagina, anus and top of the penis. It looks a bit like cottage cheese and can be painful. Treatments vary depending on its severity, and are effective. Thrush can begin to appear before your CD4 cell count falls below 200.

CMV (cytomegalovirus)
Cytomegalovirus means great cell virus. It can affect the eyes, gut, lungs and nervous system. If not treated early, it can cause very serious problems such as blindness. CMV occurs in people with very advanced HIV disease.

Treatment for CMV used to be given by intravenous injection, but more recently effective oral treatments have become available.

Cryptococcal meningitis
Cryptococcus is a fungus found in bird excrement. In humans, it usually infects the lungs, causing a chest infection, but can rapidly infect the meninges (the lining of the brain) causing fever, headache, stiff neck and

confusion. A lumbar puncture is needed to properly diagnose it. Meningitis occurs in people with very advanced HIV disease.

Different treatments are used depending on the severity of the infection, and in very severe cases these drugs can have quite severe side-effects. After recovering from meningitis, it is important to take prophylactic treatment to stop it coming back.

Cryptosporidiosis

Cryptosporidiosis, normally abbreviated to just crypto, is caused by a parasite that gets into the gut. It is normally transmitted in the water supply, or by contact with human or animal excrement. It causes watery diarrhoea, which can lead to very rapid weight loss. It can also infect the liver, causing inflammation.

Crypto often clears up by itself after a few weeks in people with less damaged immune systems. Although many drugs can be used to treat it, none are completely effective. Anti-diarrhoea and rehydration treatments are important in limiting the severity of the illness. It is also wise to see a dietitian if you get crypto, to make sure that you are getting enough nutrients from your diet.

HIV encephalopathy

This disease, sometimes called AIDS dementia complex or HIV-associated dementia, is caused by HIV's direct effects on the central nervous system. The first symptoms consist of minor changes in behaviour, coordination and concentration. Sometimes, those affected become apathetic or withdrawn. In some cases, it becomes much worse, resulting in a loss of control of movement, schizophrenia and suicidal impulses.

Many other illnesses can cause nervous or mental health problems, and HIV-associated dementia is very rare. However, it can occur in people who have very low CD4 cell counts.

The only effective treatment is anti-HIV therapy, and the success of anti-HIV treatments is the main reason why HIV-associated dementia is now so rare.

Kaposi's sarcoma (KS)

KS is a cancer which occurs most commonly on the skin, but can also affect the organs and intestines. It is thought to be caused by a type of herpes virus that is sexually transmitted. Most cases of KS in this country have been seen in gay men.

KS looks like purple, brown or black marks on the skin. These can look like bruises, bites or other infections, so a biopsy of the affected area is needed to confirm KS.

KS normally develops when you have a low CD4 cell count. The best way of treating it is to boost the immune system. Anti-HIV treatment regimens based on either protease inhibitors or NNRTIs have been shown to be equally effective at getting rid of KS. Individual lesions on the skin can be frozen off, and KS affecting the internal organs or intestines can be treated with chemotherapy or radiotherapy.

Lymphoma
This is cancer of the lymphatic system: the body's internal drainage system. It is normally seen in the lymph nodes, which swell up, but it can spread throughout the body. Symptoms include night sweats and fevers, but remember that many infections can cause these symptoms, as well as swelling of the lymph nodes.

Lymphoma has become a lot less common since effective anti-HIV treatments became available, and when it does develop, it can often be successfully treated with chemotherapy or radiotherapy.

MAI
This is caused by a bacteria similar to tuberculosis. It can be caught from soil or tap water. It only affects people with very severely damaged immune systems, when it can cause weight loss, fever and diarrhoea. If you have a very low CD4 cell count, your doctor might recommend that you take preventative treatment to stop you getting MAI. There are a number of treatments against MAI, but their success varies. As with many AIDS-defining illnesses, the best treatment is often to strengthen the immune system using anti-HIV treatments.

PCP (pneumocystis pneumonia)
PCP and tuberculosis are the two most common AIDS-defining illness in the UK. PCP affects about 200 people every year. It is a fungus that lives in the lungs and causes inflammation in a person who has a damaged immune system.

PCP can be a very dangerous infection if not treated early, so you should always tell your doctor if you have a persistent dry cough and shortness of breath. Other symptoms include fever and night sweats.

There are highly effective treatments against PCP, the most common being co-trimoxazole, but this can cause an allergic reaction. To avoid this, your doctor may desensitise you to the drug by giving you a progressively larger dose each day, over a number of days.

PCP rarely develops in people whose CD4 cell counts are above 200, the point at which you should start taking anti-HIV treatment. If your CD4 cell count is below or around 200 you should take PCP prophylaxis, even if you are taking anti-HIV treatments, until your CD4 cell count increases. PCP prophylaxis also protects against toxoplasmosis (see below).

Thrombocytopenia

This means that you have a low number of platelets in your blood - small cells that help your blood to clot. It can cause bruising and, in serious cases, internal bleeding.

As it is often caused by HIV itself, the most effective treatment is HIV therapy. It is very important not to take anti-inflammatory drugs such as ibuprofen, as they can make the condition worse and cause internal bleeding.

Toxoplasmosis

Toxoplasmosis, or 'toxo' for short, is caused by a parasite transmitted in raw or undercooked meat. Cat faeces are also a theoretical risk.

Toxo can cause cysts to form on the brain, leading to headaches, fever, drowsiness, and fits. Without treatment, these can become very severe and lead to coma.

The drug used to treated PCP, co-trimoxazole, is also effective against toxo - so the condition is very rare, partly because people who are at risk of toxo are already taking co-trimoxazole to stop them getting PCP.

Tuberculosis (TB)

TB and PCP are the two most common AIDS-defining illness seen in the UK, with around 200 cases of TB diagnosed in HIV-positive individuals each year. Worldwide, TB is the leading cause of illness and death in people with HIV.

TB is caused by a very small bacterium. It is a very serious infection and causes fever, coughing, chest pain and weight loss. Unlike nearly every other AIDS-defining illness, you can become ill with TB even when you have a relatively high CD4 cell count.

TB is treated with a combination of antibiotics, which are normally taken for six months. These have to be taken very rigorously, or you run the risk of developing multi-drug-resistant TB.

For more information on TB, you can read the free NAM booklet *HIV and TB*, which is available from HIV clinics or can be downloaded from www.aidsmap.com.

Illnesses in the age of anti-HIV treatment - cancers

Anti-HIV treatments have brought longer and healthier lives for many people with HIV. Indeed, side-effects of treatment are the most likely cause of ill-health in HIV-positive people now, and in many cases these either lessen with time or can be controlled.

However, around 500 people a year in the UK develop an AIDS-defining illness, and around 400 people die every year because of HIV-related causes. Although illnesses such as PCP and TB still cause illness and even death in people with HIV, it seems that cancers and coinfection with hepatitis B and/or hepatitis C are becoming more common as causes of illness and death in people with HIV.

Kaposi's sarcoma and non-Hodgkin's lymphoma have become rarer since the introduction of effective anti-HIV treatment, but still cause illness and death in people with HIV. Often, these people have very weak immune systems, but there have been cases of these cancers developing in people who are taking HIV treatments and have good CD4 cell counts.

Other cancers that are not regarded as AIDS-defining conditions appear to have become more common in HIV-positive people since effective anti-HIV treatment became available. There is no evidence that anti-HIV drugs cause these cancers. The increased rates of some cancers seen in people with HIV since the introduction of HIV treatment have come about because people are living longer, and not dying of other illnesses.

Anal cancer

Anal cancer is emerging as a health concern, particularly for HIV-positive gay men. Human papilloma virus (HPV), the cause of genital and anal warts, is the underlying cause of anal cancer, and anti-HIV drugs are not effective against HPV. There has been a very slight increase in the amount of anal cancer seen in people with HIV since the introduction of anti-HIV treatments. Doctors think that this could be because HIV-positive people are living longer.

Before cancer develops, pre-cancerous lesions, called AIN (anal intraepithelial neoplasia), form. These are graded AIN I, AIN II, and AIN III according to severity. It takes a long time for AIN to progress to anal cancer. In some cases, AIN may be removed surgically.

Anal cancer is treated aggressively, with a combination of chemotherapy and radiotherapy. Sometimes, surgery is also needed, and the overall cure rate is about 60%.

Some HIV clinics are looking at the value of screening people with HPV in their anus or rectum for AIN. This involves using a test very similar to the PAP smear used to detect pre-cancerous cervical cells in women. Although these tests aren't 100% accurate, the earlier AIN is detected, the greater the chance of effective treatment.

Lung cancer

People with HIV seem to be at increased risk of developing lung cancer. It's very rare, however, and the outcome is no worse in people with HIV than it is in those without HIV. In one study, all the HIV-positive people who developed lung cancer were smokers.

Testicular cancer

There's some evidence to suggest that testicular cancer is more common in HIV-positive men. The reason for this isn't known. If you notice a lump in your testicles you should see a doctor as soon as possible. Treatment works just as well in HIV-positive men as in HIV-negative men. The sooner treatment is provided the better.

Cervical cancer

Since the mid-1990s, cervical cancer has been an AIDS-defining condition. Doctors have noticed an increase in the incidence of cervical cancer since effective HIV treatment became available. It's important for HIV-positive women to have regular PAP smears.

Liver cancer

For information on liver cancer, see the section on *Illnesses in the age of anti-HIV treatment - hepatitis.*

Illnesses in the age of anti-HIV treatment - hepatitis

Coinfection with hepatitis B virus or/and hepatitis C virus is increasingly becoming a cause of illness in people with HIV. Both these viruses affect the liver, can make you very ill and can be fatal.

Hepatitis B

Hepatitis B virus (often known as HBV) is an infection that can cause severe or even fatal damage to the liver. Long-term infection with hepatitis B can cause liver cancer, and rates of liver cancer in people with HIV are elevated

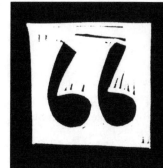

because of hepatitis B and hepatitis C. Hepatitis B is quite common in some of the communities affected by HIV in the UK, as it can be contracted in the same ways as HIV, particularly through contact with blood, semen or vaginal fluid, and from mother to baby.

You should be tested soon after your diagnosis for hepatitis B, to see if you have been infected with the virus and are a carrier. A vaccine is available to protect you against hepatitis B. If you are uninfected, and a test shows that you do not have natural immunity against it, you should be vaccinated.

If you are coinfected with hepatitis B, doctors will regularly monitor your liver function using blood tests. Ultrasound examinations may also be performed, particularly if your liver shows signs of damage.

Treatments are available for hepatitis B, and three drugs have been licensed. These are alpha-interferon, the anti-HIV drug 3TC (lamivudine) and adefovir (*Hepsera*). Tenfovir (*Viread*) and FTC (emtricitabine, *Emtriva*) are also effective against hepatitis B, but have not yet been formally licensed for the treatment of HIV/hepatitis B coinfection. Tenfovir and FTC are available in a combined pill called *Truvada*.

Having hepatitis B is not thought to make HIV progress faster. Anti-HIV drugs can be used safely and effectively in people with hepatitis B. However, when some people start anti-HIV treatment, they experience a short-term flare-up of hepatitis B. This is because the immune system is getting stronger and is fighting hepatitis B. Some doctors try to stop these flare-ups happening by starting treatment for HIV and hepatitis B at the same time. Some anti-HIV drugs can cause abnormal liver function, including ritonavir (*Norvir*), indinavir (*Crixivan*), nevirapine (*Viracept*), AZT (*Retrovir*) and ddI and should be used with caution if you have hepatitis B.

British treatment guidelines recommend that if you have hepatitis B and HIV, your anti-HIV treatment should include a drug that is effective against hepatitis B. These are 3TC, tenofovir and FTC. Some doctors think that a combination including 3TC and tenofovir is a very effective treatment for both hepatitis B and HIV.

Because of the risk of developing drug resistance, you should only take anti-HIV drugs to treat hepatitis B as part of an anti-HIV treatment regimen. If you are going to take treatment just for hepatitis B (and not for HIV), you should take alpha interferon or adefovir.

Hepatitis C

Hepatitis C is transmitted through blood, and the sharing of injecting equipment is the most common route of hepatitis C transmission in the UK.

Many people also contracted hepatitis C before blood screening procedures and sterilisation were introduced, and 95% of people with haemophilia and HIV in the UK are also coinfected with hepatitis C.

The sexual transmission of hepatitis C is now an issue of concern. It used to be thought that this was very rare. However, there have been recent reports of increasing numbers of gay men testing positive for hepatitis C. Many of these men are HIV-positive and their only risk activity was unprotected anal sex. Sexual activity that carries a risk of contact with blood, such as fisting, seems to have a particular risk of hepatitis C transmission.

Mother-to-baby transmission of hepatitis C is thought to be uncommon, but the risk is increased if the mother is also HIV-positive. A high hepatitis C viral load also increases the risk that a mother will pass on hepatitis C to her baby, and, as with HIV, a caesarean delivery reduces the risk.

Very few people experience symptoms when they are first infected with hepatitis C. When they do occur, symptoms include jaundice, diarrhoea, and feeling sick. In the longer term, about 50% of people with hepatitis C will experience some symptoms. The most common ones are feeling generally unwell, extreme tiredness, weight loss, depression, and intolerance of fatty food and alcohol.

Although a small proportion of people infected with hepatitis C clear the infection naturally, about 85% will go on to develop chronic hepatitis C. About a third of people will develop severe liver disease within 15 to 25 years.

The severity of disease can be affected by the strain of hepatitis C you are infected with. Men, people who drink alcohol, people who are infected with hepatitis C when they are already into middle age, and people with HIV seem to experience faster hepatitis C disease progression.

Hepatitis C can cause liver fibrosis and cirrhosis. This damages the liver to such an extent that it cannot work properly, causing jaundice, internal bleeding, and swelling of the abdomen. Chronic infection with hepatitis C can cause liver cancer. Liver cancer is especially likely to happen in people with cirrhosis, particularly if they drink heavily.

There's also some evidence that smoking can speed up the rate of cirrhosis and increase the risk of liver cancer.

Liver cancer is difficult to treat, and often surgery is the only option. Small tumours can be removed, but there's a high chance of them recurring. Chemotherapy is not effective against liver cancer.

You should be tested soon after your diagnosis with HIV to see if you are also infected with hepatitis C. Unlike hepatitis B, there is no vaccine against hepatitis C, and if you are in a group at high risk of infection with hepatitis C, it's recommended that you should have frequent tests to see if you have been infected.

A test is also available to measure hepatitis C viral load (PCR). Unlike the HIV viral load test, this is not an indicator of when to start treatment. However, it is used to show how effective treatment for hepatitis C is and how long it should continue for.

Liver function tests can give an indication of the extent to which hepatitis C has damaged your liver. Liver ultrasounds and liver biopsies may also be used.

It seems that people coinfected with HIV and hepatitis C are more likely to develop liver disease than people who are only infected with hepatitis C.

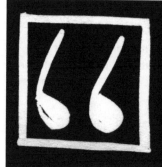

I went to my consultant because of a cough that wouldn't go away. After a while she said, "I think you have a virus." I looked at her with a smile on my face and said, "Oh really, tell me about it!" We both cracked-up laughing.

positive voice

However, hepatitis C does not seem to increase your risk of becoming ill due to HIV, developing or dying of AIDS, or responding less well to anti-HIV treatment.

Anti-HIV treatment can be used safely and effectively if you are coinfected with HIV and hepatitis C. However, you may be at greater risk of experiencing the liver side-effects which some anti-HIV drugs can cause, and you and your doctor should have this in mind when selecting which anti-HIV drugs to take. It also seems to be the case that people coinfected with HIV and hepatitis C are at greater risk of developing some of the metabolic disorders which anti-HIV drugs can cause (particularly insulin resistance and diabetes).

Drugs are available for the treatment of hepatitis C and you should receive your treatment and care from doctors who are expert in the treatment of both HIV and hepatitis C. This may mean that as well as seeing an HIV doctor, you may also need to see a specialist liver doctor.

Before you start treatment for hepatitis C, it is important to know which strain, or genotype, of hepatitis C you have been infected with, as this can predict your response to treatment and the amount of time you will need to take treatment for. There are several hepatitis C genotypes. Type 1 is most common in the UK, and unfortunately responds least well to the currently available treatments for hepatitis C.

Unlike anti-HIV treatment, treatment for hepatitis C is not lifelong. It consists of 24 or 48 weeks of treatment, and the length of treatment you receive will depend on the hepatitis C genotype you are infected with. A test after 12 weeks of treatment can predict if you are going to respond to treatment.

Drugs available for the treatment of hepatitis C. These are pegylated interferon and ribavirin. Treatment with a combination of pegylated interferon and ribavirin is the standard treatment, as it produces better results and is recommended by British HIV doctors.

If you have a CD4 cell count above 200, then the aim of hepatitis C treatment is to eradicate infection with hepatitis C completely. Although over 50% of people who are only infected with hepatitis C achieve this, the response rate is much lower in people with HIV.

Other aims of treatment include normalising liver function, reducing liver inflammation and reducing further damage to the liver. If you are ill because of HIV, then the aim of hepatitis C treatment is likely to focus on improving your tolerance of anti-HIV drugs, reducing the risk of death from liver problems and improving your overall quality of life.

Hepatitis C treatment can have unpleasant side-effects, including temperature, joint pain, weight loss, nausea and vomiting and depression. Other side-effects include disturbances in blood chemistry.

If you are taking ribavirin you should not take ddI (didanosine, *Videx*), d4T (stavudine, *Zerit*) or tenofovir (*Viread*), because of the risk of very serious side-effects, including pancreatitis and lactic acidosis. Nor should ribavirin and AZT (zidovudine, *Retrovir*) be taken together, because of the risk of anaemia.

The infection which is the greatest risk to your health should be treated first. If you have a good CD4 cell count and are not ill because of HIV, then you should be given the chance to start hepatitis C treatment before starting HIV drugs. However, if your CD4 cell count is below 200, or is rapidly falling, or you are ill because of HIV, then you should start HIV treatment first.

Liver transplants
An increasing number of liver transplants are being performed on people with HIV who are coinfected with hepatitis B or C.

You are most likely to be considered for a liver transplant if HIV hasn't done too much damage to your immune system, or you have responded well to anti-HIV drugs, and have a good CD4 cell count and a low viral load.

Liver transplants seem to be just as successful in people coinfected with HIV and hepatitis B or C as in people who are just infected with either hepatitis B or C. Studies have found that HIV-positive people are just as likely as HIV-negative transplant recipients to be alive three years after receiving their new liver.

Organ transplant is a very specialist medical skill, and there's a chance that the hospital where you receive your HIV care may not be a centre with expertise in this area. This could mean that you are referred to another hospital.

If you have a successful liver transplant, you will need to take medication to stop your body rejecting your new liver for the rest of your life. You'll still have to take your anti-HIV medication as well.

Further reading

- NAM factsheets: *Anal cancer, Blood problems, Cervical cancer, Dementia, Diarrhoea, Fatigue, Genital warts, Hepatitis B, Hepatitis C, Immunisations, Kaposi's sarcoma, Liver, Mouth problems, Nausea and vomiting, Non-Hodgkin's lymphoma, Pain, PCP, Preventing infections, Skin problems, Sight problems, Tuberculosis, Weight loss* and *Winter viral illnesses.*

- *HIV and hepatitis, HIV and sex* and *HIV and TB,* booklets in the information for HIV-positive people series produced by NAM.

- 'Symptoms and illnesses' in NAM's *HIV and AIDS Treatments Directory.*

- 'Hepatitis coinfection' in NAM's *HIV and AIDS Reference Manual.*

- *The risks of hepatitis B,* and *The risks of hepatitis C,* booklets produced by the Terrence Higgins Trust.

Headaches
by Martin

In October 2000 I arrived in the UK from Zimbabwe. I went to live in Bristol with my then partner. Things went okay, and I went to college and then was granted a work visa and right to remain in the UK.

Since childhood, I've had headaches, and in the spring of 2005 I went to see my GP because of them. My GP was concerned about my headaches and said I should go for an HIV test. An appointment was also made for me to see a specialist about my headaches.

My HIV test was positive and my headaches intensified. I went to work the day after I found out I had HIV, but the day after my headaches were so bad I had to spend the day in bed. The day after that I was admitted to hospital.

I more or less passed out as soon as they admitted me and I'm not really sure what happened for the next three weeks. Initially tuberculosis was suspected, but eventually they diagnosed cryptococcal meningitis and I was treated for it. I was in hospital for three months.

I started antiretroviral treatment, my CD4 cell count was very low at only 72. After starting HIV treatment I had strange dreams. My doctor explained that these were a side-effect of the efavirenz as I was taking as part of my anti-HIV combination.

Even though I did not feel very well I was discharged from hospital and went home. The only support I received was from a care assistant who did my shopping for me.

Soon I became ill again and spent another three months in hospital. I was very unstable on my feet, and I had loads of tests, including lumbar punctures which were very uncomfortable and an operation to remove fluid from my brain.

When I was discharged from hospital, I was provided with support from a nurse who visited me in my home and from a social worker. I've also received support from THT in Bristol and I am now a volunteer there.

My anti-HIV treatment is working and my CD4 cell count has been steadily improving. I make sure that I always take my medicines so that they work properly.

It's the bigots I feel sorry for

I was infected by HIV in New York in 1984 but diagnosed in 1985 while at home in Scotland for the summer holidays. It was a nightmare. I went back to New York and it took me a year to come to terms with it.

In August 1995 I became very ill and within a week I was back in the UK and admitted to the Chelsea and Westminster Hospital in London. I was only there for one night and my mother was there with me. The next day I was discharged and we went to my aunt and uncle's house in Surrey. They asked us to leave next day. My fever was 105 and I was so frail I had to be helped onto the train back to Scotland by the guard.

1996 was my worst year and my health was never better than "so so." In September, after a stay in a hospice, I was popping 50 pills a day. My left eye was damaged by CMV, but thankfully I could still see.

In late 1998 I started to become unwell again and by March 1999 I was admitted to the Western General Hospital in Edinburgh where I received excellent care and support.

But the side-effects of the 50 or so pills a day I was taking were so bad I had to stop taking them.

My treatment changed and I was now taking a total of six pills in equal doses in the morning and at night.

My weight increased from only nine stone when I was admitted to hospital in the Spring of 1999 to 13 stone by the end of 1999. I began swimming, playing tennis, dancing, going out and enjoying life.

Then everything changed. I started getting abusive phone calls and was called a poof on the High Street. But by far the worst thing happened in December 2000. My Mum was recovering from a stroke at the time, it was Christmas week. There was a knock at the door. Nobody was there, but somebody had scratched 'AIDS' on the bonnet of the car.

I was since diagnosed with cancer - thankfully I recovered - and am my Mum's full-time carer.

But I'm still targeted by small-minded bigots. I was recently sent a very nasty letter saying I was a "scum bag" who bled the system and should either leave town or just lay down and die. The police are investigating it, but I doubt anything will come of it.

I get on with my life, making the most of the health that I have. I travel and recently took my Mum to Italy for her 80th birthday.

My Mum is very supportive, and most of the 3,000 people who live in my town are fine. It's just those few small-minded bigots. You have to ask yourself what have they got in their life? I feel sorry for them, I really do.

No bed of roses

What I would like to know is: why is being HIV-positive so often portrayed as being a bed of roses these days?

I was diagnosed in 1994 at which time I had already been infected for about ten years. My CD4 count was zero, and viral load tests weren't being used as part of routine HIV care yet. My diagnosis came after a year of PCP pneumonia treated as asthma. There has been a steady stream of 'afflictions' ever since. Some caused by the virus itself, some by the anti-viral drugs.

First to go was my sense of balance. My gait became unsteady. I joined a drug trial that gave me heart failure (thought to be terminal). That put paid to my ability to walk, especially after vacuolar myelopathy ate away at my spine. I've been permanently in a wheel chair ever since. The protease inhibitor indinavir came along and saved my life. However, this was at a cost. It caused diabetes and kidney stones. My right kidney, to this day, is still a cause for concern.

I also have a permanent urethral catheter which gets in the way sexually. I've also pancreatitis, anaemia (requiring several blood transfusions), anal cancer requiring extensive surgery leading to a permanent colostomy, disfiguring lipodystrophy and liver disease which has caused serious bleeding problems.

My latest, and worst, problem has been caused by intestinal adhesions brought on by abdominal surgery. This leads to occasional hospitalisations to treat blockage of my bowel. It is as good as untreatable and causes me significant discomfort and pain on a daily basis. I must eat an insipid, fibre-free diet. I suffer from alternating bouts of constipation and floods of diarrhoea. Some days my belly is so swollen I can't even squeeze in sips of water. On these days I eat nothing at all, which would be pointless as I vomit a few times a day.

Each of these can be glibly rhymed off as a list of medical conditions but they each cause physical discomfort, self-image issues and real life practical difficulties. For example, how do you take medicine twice daily with food when you can't eat for days at a time?

My life feels fragile and precious. You have to appreciate life, preserve it and never take it for granted, whether living with HIV or not.

TB - my experiences
by Nick

This might sound odd, but I was really shocked when I became seriously ill because of HIV. I was even more shocked when it turned out to be tuberculosis.

I was diagnosed with HIV in the early 1990s. At that time, there was only one drug - AZT - and I was sure that HIV would kill me within about ten years. Well, by the summer of 1994 nothing had happened. My CD4 cell count was just as high as the day I was diagnosed and, to be honest, I felt healthier than ever. It really felt like a kind of phony war - the regular clinic visits for tests were nothing more than a minor inconvenience, and I even dared to think that I might be one of the handful of individuals I'd read about who remained healthy with HIV for years on end.

With these thoughts in mind, I didn't pay too much attention to a newspaper report I read about the first increase in tuberculosis cases in the UK since vaccination, effective antibiotics, and improved housing and nutrition came along after the last war. I wasn't even concerned when I read that many of the cases involved people with HIV. I also felt reassured because I'd had a tuberculosis vaccine as a teenager. And on top of it all, I just felt so healthy.

How wrong I was.

The first symptom was a mild, dull pain in my lower right chest. I felt certain it was just a pulled muscle and carried on as normal. I wasn't alarmed when I started waking up in the middle of the right with a light sweat on my forehead. It was summer, after all. And I also found an easy explanation, simple tiredness, for the severe breathlessness I experienced on my 16-mile Sunday run.

It was, however, much harder to explain away the temperature of 104 degrees I awoke with the following Monday. That something was seriously the matter was confirmed at the hospital by a chest x-ray showing a mass of fluid on my right lung - exactly where the pain had been for the past few months. Initially, I was treated for bacterial pneumonia. PCP pneumonia was ruled out as my CD4 cell count was about 500. I didn't get any better. Further tests over the next few days, which involved draining over two litres of fluid from my lung and a biopsy, confirmed that I had tuberculosis.

How could I have got tuberculosis? I asked myself. The answer was simple, I was HIV-positive and even the very mild immune damage I'd experienced was enough to undermine whatever protection my childhood vaccination offered and leave me vulnerable to infection with tuberculosis and the development of disease.

I was physically and emotionally wrecked. In the space of a fortnight, I lost a stone in weight and became very weak. I had to rely on my partner and friends to undertake household tasks for me. But just as severe was the emotional impact. The combination of anti-tuberculosis drugs quickly controlled my symptoms and, as I was careful to take every dose of my six-month course of treatment, I was completely cured. Although my CD4 cell count fell by about a half to 250, within six months I was able to run just as often and as far as before, with only the very occasional twinge of pain in my chest to remind me of the scarring caused by the tuberculosis.

But the emotional impact was much more permanent. I realised just how serious HIV was, and accepted for the first time that I'd probably have a series of severe illness over the coming years before a premature and inevitable death. As I result, I left work and planned as pleasant as possible a retirement for my last few years of life.

It hasn't quite worked out like that, thanks to the anti-HIV drugs I've been taking since 1998. But in summer 1994, effective anti-HIV treatments, and the hope that they've brought for me, were a very long way away.

Paul
living with HIV and hepatitis C and haemophilia

For most people, coping with HIV is enough of a problem in itself, but when you throw in a lifetime disorder such as haemophilia, and then add hepatitis C virus to the list, it does complicate things.

I was born with haemophilia, so it's something I have known all my life, and something that I have grown up coping with. I've never known anything different. The damage to my joints caused by internal bleeding has left me with chronic arthritis, which impairs my mobility and causes daily pain.

I was diagnosed as HTLV-3 positive, as HIV was known in 1985, and given little hope of a future, along with over 1200 others with haemophilia in the UK. There was no pre- or post-test counselling offered and very little advice. The only thing I was told for certain was that I wouldn't have long to live.

In 1992, I was told I had also become hepatitis C virus positive, through the same route of infection as my HIV -

contaminated Factor VIII, the treatment I took to prevent internal bleeding.

I was told that HIV would cause my death many years before hepatitis C would be a problem and advised not to worry about it.

By 1998 I had numerous HIV-related illnesses, a very low CD4 count and an extremely worrying increasing viral load. I started antiretroviral therapy, which was a turning point for me, not only in addressing my HIV, but also in contemplating the effects of my other conditions.

Protease inhibitors have been shown to cause increased internal bleeding in people with haemophilia, so they were not an option. I was also concerned about the effects any drugs would have on my liver and the impact they may have on my hepatitis C. My hardest task at the time was finding information about co-infection. The HIV organisations knew about HIV and the hepatitis organisations about hepatitis but neither seemed to know much about both viruses in combination.

I started treatment with a regimen of nevirapine and Combivir, which have luckily worked well - I am still on the same regimen six years later. However, four months into this medication, alarm bells were ringing about nevirapine and hepatic failure. My liver function test results had escalated since I began HIV treatment and I was in turmoil, worried that although one set of drugs were working well against the HIV, they might be causing increased hepatic problems. Again I struggled to find information, running back and forth between two hospitals and three different consultants - who never met each other.

Eventually, my liver function test results reduced. They were still abnormally high, but were now at a level that wasn't scaring me, or my doctors, too much.

The HIV drugs were working, and for the first time in 15 years I actually thought I might have a future. The advent of pegylated interferon and ribavarin gave me hope for treating my hepatitis C. I wanted to start treatment and agreed with my doctors to start a trial. I had weighed up the consequences, read as much as I could about what to expect and talked to other people who had undergone hepatitis C treatment. I discussed with my hepatologist and my HIV consultant, as well as both sets of pharmacists, what options were available and what possible HAART regimen changes could be made if needed.

I told most of my family and friends that I was to start hepatitis C treatment and planned my life so that I had time to cope with side-effects. By the time the trial was due to start, the hospital ethics committee had decided to exclude people with HIV. This was a devastating blow at the time, and didn't help my relationships with my doctors. The same hospital that had infected me with both viruses wouldn't give me the opportunity to try and treat one because of the other.

I heard many stories about the horrific side-effects that some people were having on this medication and by the time pegylated interferon was licensed, I had my reservations about trying treatment. By now I had more questions. I have hepatitis C-genotype one, which is the hardest to treat, needing twelve months' of therapy and still giving the poorest results. I knew that AZT and ribavarin were causing problems for the majority, and now I was scared about changing my HIV treatment regimen because it was working so well for my HIV. I didn't want to jeopardise the success of my HIV therapy, to have twelve months of hell and only a 25% chance of success if I endured the treatment. It all seemed too much of a gamble.

All my illnesses concern me. My arthritis hurts daily, I have to inject factor 8 when needed, my twice-daily visit to my pill box reminds me, as do the nausea and the night sweats, of my HIV - and my liver throbs at times. I don't know what the future holds, but I am hoping that hepatitis C medication improves before my liver deteriorates. It's a big gamble, but the last 20 years have also been a gamble, against all odds. I have been crossing my fingers and trying to stay informed along the way, and I will continue to do so.

The luxury of hypochondriacs
by Caroline Guinness

That anxious look I get from loved ones is very hard to take, and all I want to do is reassure them that everything will be all right. Complicated, isn't it?!

When I was first diagnosed with HIV, I felt very isolated. I had a gay friend with AIDS but I did not tell him about my diagnosis as I didn't want to worry him. He was very ill at the time and I felt my health was OK - the last thing I wanted to do was give him something else to cope with, so I looked after him and forgot about my own HIV.

The few friends I told at the time were shocked and very concerned about my health. Again, I did not want to worry them, so I did not discuss what I was going through. I became aware that I could no longer whinge about any aches, pains, colds or any other 'normal, everyday maladies', because to them it represented something far more serious.

I coped for a while by just being in complete denial, but I began to feel isolated and longed to be able to speak freely about my situation, longed to meet other women in the same situation as myself.

I met other positive women for the first time at a support group. It made an enormous difference, the relief of being able to talk, knowing they were feeling the same things, made me feel 'normal' for the first time in ages. I went on to run support groups and discovered, again and again, that no matter what the cultural differences might be, we all had basically the same problems - the main one being how to cope with our HIV status.

Then I started to realise that my (HIV-negative) friends were treating me differently. I had always offered a shoulder to any one of them who needed it. But what I began to find was that even if I could see that they were going through a difficult time, they did not seem to want to talk to me about it. Over dinner one night, a good girlfriend, having consumed rather too much alcohol, informed me that she did not feel she could confide her problems to me as she felt mine were so much bigger than hers...BINGO...I understood what was going on.

I tried tell my friends that their problems were relevant and of course I still wanted to be confided in and asked for friendly advice. Whenever I said this, I was always greeted with `but I don't want to worry you'. Luckily, as the years have gone by they have become used to my HIV, and our relationships carry on as normal. I never did want to be treated differently. Having said that though, I have learned to never complain about any illness unless I know it is really serious... and even then I play it down.

My circle of HIV-positive friends grew and I felt I had a great balance. Every now and then, I would meet up with my peers, have a few drinks and be able to talk about anything related to our status.

Since moving to the country, I have had little contact with my HIV-positive friends. One night last week I met up with a group of friends, one of whom was positive. It felt like manna from heaven, and without realising it, he and I immediately fell into `HIV speak' and forgot about everyone else at the table - we could talk about our `aches and pains' and not worry each other.

I think when you are suffering from a life-threatening illness you do not want to tell people about your everyday symptoms. I have realised that it is a luxury for healthy people to complain about their health. The usual advice to them is along the lines of: "Oh don't worry, it is only a cold/flu, everyone's going down with it, have some Lemsip, you'll be fine." The only people who seem able to say this to me are others in the same situation... who are also HIV-positive.

So to any healthy hypochondriacs reading this, do not feel guilty, you have a luxury I really miss. To moan and not be taken seriously... yes, please.

This first appeared in issue 87 of Positive Nation, February 2003. Many thanks to both Caroline and Positive Nation for giving permission to reprint it.

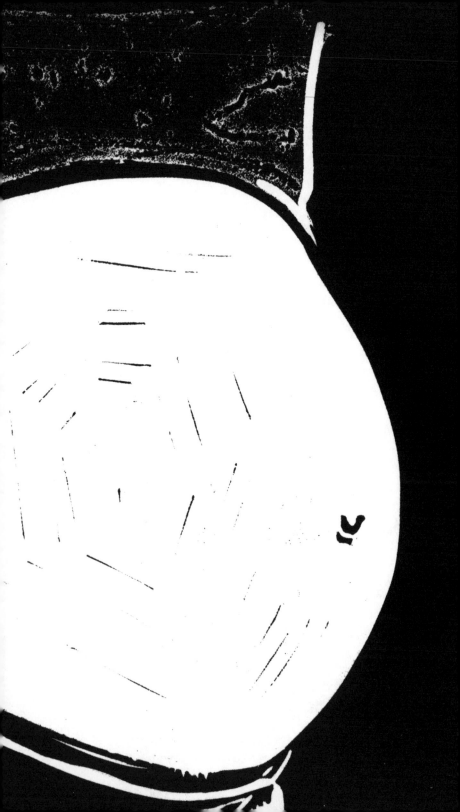

Mother-to-baby transmission of HIV

In this chapter you'll find information on

How to prevent mother-to-baby
transmission of HIV.

How anti-HIV drugs should be used to
prevent mother-to-baby transmission.

The best mode of delivery to prevent
mother-to-baby transmission.

The importance of not breastfeeding.

Two women write about their experiences of
pregnancy and measures to prevent
mother-to-baby transmission.

An HIV-positive woman can pass on HIV to her baby during pregnancy, or during delivery, or by breastfeeding.

Anti-HIV treatment can, however, greatly reduce the risks of a woman passing on HIV to her baby. Having a caesarean rather than a vaginal delivery can reduce the risks even further. The exclusive use of formula feed is strongly recommended for all babies with HIV-positive mothers in the UK. Using these methods, it's possible to reduce the risk of mother-to-baby transmission of HIV from about one in four to less than one in a hundred.

A number of factors can make it more likely that a woman will pass on HIV to her baby. These include:

- Being ill because of HIV.
- Having a high HIV viral load and a low CD4 cell count.
- Waters breaking four hours or more before delivery.
- Having an untreated sexually transmitted infection at the time of delivery.
- Using recreational drugs, particularly injected drugs, during pregnancy.
- Having a vaginal delivery (rather than a caesarean delivery) if HIV viral load is detectable.
- Having a difficult delivery, requiring, for example the use of forceps.
- Breastfeeding.

Preventing mother-to-baby transmission with anti-HIV drugs

Introduction

Taking anti-HIV drugs can dramatically reduce the risk of you passing on HIV to your baby. There are two different ways in which these drugs act.

First, they reduce your viral load so your baby is exposed to less HIV while in the womb and during birth. The aim of HIV treatment is to get, and keep, your viral load below 50. This is often referred to as an undetectable viral load.

Second, anti-HIV drugs may cross the placenta and enter your baby's body, preventing the virus from ever taking hold. Newborn babies are given a short course of anti-HIV drugs after they are born when their mother is known to be HIV-positive.

Two drugs have been shown to be very effective at preventing mother-to-baby transmission of HIV in the second of these ways. These are the nucleoside analogue (NRTI) AZT (zidovudine, *Retrovir*) and the non-nucleoside (NNRTI) nevirapine (*Viramune*). It's also likely that other drugs are also very effective, but these haven't been tested as extensively.

The ways in which anti-HIV drugs are used (on their own or in combination with other anti-HIV drugs) will depend on the damage HIV has done to your immune system, and the point in your pregnancy when your HIV was diagnosed.

In the UK, and other countries where there is easy access to anti-HIV drugs, nevirapine should not be used by itself (as monotherapy) to prevent mother-to-baby transmission of HIV, because resistance to the drug can rapidly develop if it is used in this way. Using it alone would limit your ability to benefit from nevirapine or related drugs in the future, when you may need them to protect your own health. Nor should nevirapine be used in combination with other HIV drugs if you have a CD4 cell count above 250, as there is a risk of potentially dangerous side-effects.

In good health?

If you have a CD4 cell count that is high enough to protect you from becoming ill because of HIV, and a low HIV viral load, and you are not ill because of HIV, then UK doctors recommend that you should receive treatment with AZT during the final three months (third trimester) of pregnancy. You will also be given an intravenous dose of AZT during labour, and will need to have a caesarean rather than a vaginal delivery.

Another option is to take a short course of three anti-HIV drugs during the last few months of pregnancy in order to get your viral load below 50. You will then have the option of having a planned vaginal delivery.

Your baby will need to take AZT syrup for four to six weeks.

High viral load, low CD4 cell count?

If HIV has damaged your immune system, meaning that you are vulnerable to infections, or if you have a high viral load, then you are advised to take three anti-HIV drugs, including the NRTIs AZT and 3TC, the NNRTI nevirapine or a protease inhibitor. You should not take nevirapine if your CD4 cell count is above 250. The higher your viral load, the earlier in pregnancy you will need to start taking treatment. If your viral load is still above 50 before delivery, then you will need to have a caesarean delivery. However, a viral load below 50 should mean that you have the option of a planned vaginal delivery.

Your baby will need to take four to six weeks of AZT syrup.

Already on treatment?

If you become pregnant whilst taking anti-HIV drugs that are successfully suppressing your viral load, you are recommended to continue taking them. You will need to have a special scan at week 20 of your pregnancy, called an anomaly scan, to see if your baby is developing with abnormalities.

Your baby will need to take four to six weeks of AZT syrup.

Diagnosed late in pregnancy?

If you are diagnosed with HIV very late during pregnancy (week 32 or later), then you will need to start taking a combination of three anti-HIV drugs immediately. These should be AZT, 3TC and nevirapine (unless your CD4 cell count is above 250, in which case nevirapine should be replaced with a protease inhibitor). These drugs are able to rapidly pass across the placenta into your baby.

Your baby will need to take four to six weeks of AZT syrup.

Diagnosed during delivery or afterwards?

If you find out you have HIV during delivery, or just after, then you should be given a dose of AZT by injection and oral doses of AZT and nevirapine. Your baby will also need to take a triple combination of anti-HIV drugs.

Safety of treatment to prevent mother-to-baby transmission of HIV

There's some evidence of a slightly increased risk of having a premature or low birth-weight baby if a mother takes anti-HIV drugs, particularly a protease inhibitor, during pregnancy. However, this is a controversial issue and there's also evidence showing that protease inhibitors do not cause premature birth.

Preventing mother-to-baby transmission of HIV

Delivery

The risk of you passing on HIV to your baby is reduced if it is delivered using a planned surgical delivery. This is called an 'elective caesarean' and is scheduled to take place in the 38th week of pregnancy, but will be performed sooner if labour begins early. Taking anti-HIV drugs during a caesarean delivery reduces the risk of you passing on HIV to your baby to very low levels. However, as with all surgery, a caesarean delivery carries some risk, and these should be fully discussed with you before you give your consent to the procedure.

You are strongly recommended to have a caesarean if you have a detectable viral load, or if the only anti-HIV drug you took during pregnancy was AZT.

If your viral load has been consistently undetectable during pregnancy then you should be able to have a managed vaginal birth. This means that your doctors and midwife will make sure that your labour doesn't last too long and will take action to reduce the risk of you passing on HIV to your baby.

Infant feeding

The risk of you passing on HIV to your baby by breastfeeding can be as high as one in eight. In the UK and other countries where safe alternatives to breastfeeding are available, you are strongly recommended to feed your baby using formula feed from birth. Detailed advice and support on how to do this is available from your medical services and you should ask for help if you have difficulties meeting the cost.

Further reading

- NAM factsheets, *Mother-to-baby transmission, Pregnancy and conception,* and *Sperm washing.*

- *Anti-HIV drugs, HIV and children, HIV and women,* and *HIV therapy* booklets in the information for HIV-positive people series produced by NAM.

- 'HIV transmission' in NAM's *HIV and AIDS Reference Manual.*

- 'Anti-HIV therapy - options during pregnancy' in NAM's *HIV and AIDS Treatments Directory.*

- *Starting a family* leaflet produced by the Terrence Higgins Trust.

Matilda

I found out about my HIV status when I was 16 weeks pregnant. After I had an HIV test, I had counselling with the midwife. I told her of feeling utter disbelief about my situation and fear of how I was going to break the news to my partner. Yet, when I finally told my partner, he turned out to be understanding and supportive. I also encouraged him to take an HIV test, and he agreed, and fortunately he was negative. Since that time we have practiced safe sex.

At the same time, I told my HIV doctor and my midwife that I accepted their advice to start on early HIV treatment because I wanted to minimise the risk of infecting my unborn baby. The midwife told me that it is best if you don't breastfeed and that if you want you can have a caesarean section. I agreed with this, as by doing so you can greatly reduce the risk of infecting the baby. I also told my HIV doctor that I wanted my baby, when it was born, to take the anti-HIV medicine, AZT. Fortunately, I had a very healthy baby at the end.

I think that it is very important for pregnant African women to take an HIV test and if found positive, to start early treatment and accept other medical interventions which can help protect your unborn baby from HIV. My little girl is now four and half years old and she is negative. Thank God for that.

This testimony was first published on the Positively Women website. Thanks to the author and Positively Women for giving permission to reprint it here.

Bun in the oven

I've gone and got myself knocked up. Got myself into trouble, bun in the oven, all the clichés of pregnancy that good Catholic (unmarried) girls should avoid. Pregnant and HIV-positive; a state that ten years ago would have been met with effusions of pity and foreboding. So how do I feel? Pretty good, actually.

I would love to take the moral high ground and claim that my pregnancy was planned with SAS precision and facilitated by a gleaming, sterile, turkey-baster. But I'd be lying. More like a one-off act of Easter abandon, probably brought on by the heady excess of too many chocolate eggs. I suppose I could be held up as a harsh example to teenage girls in convent school - you only need to do it once to get pregnant. Okay, I may have done the deed many more times than once, but it was the one unprotected time and BANG, up the duff. Not bad for a 35-year-old with geriatric ovaries hurtling towards menopause.

I found out I was enceinte in Geneva, attending a conference. I did a wee on the pregnancy stick in my hotel room, expecting the result to be negative, but a faint blue line on the stick appeared, screaming: "You've got a bun in the oven, Girlfriend!"

Reeling, I picked up the phone and called the first person who came to mind at midnight - my HIV doctor. He was wonderfully reassuring and congratulatory, despite his patient from Hell calling hysterically in the middle of the night. He reassured me that the risk of transmission to the baby was less than 1% as I had an undetectable viral load and, more surprisingly, that I did not need to change my medication. My blind panic gradually changed into pleasure (with just the tiniest hint of fear).

My partner was initially paralysed with shock but has become rather pleasantly supportive and even turns a blind eye to my slovenly slothfulness.

The first few months of pregnancy haven't been too bad. I haven't been sick, despite the fact that in my previous two pregnancies I chucked up for England every day. I have been feeling exhausted and have fallen asleep a couple of times at my desk. Mild pregnancy stress-incontinence doesn't go so well with the hay fever season and sneezing all day, but at least it's encouraging me to do my pelvic floor exercises.

I kept my pregnancy very quiet until I had my twelve-week scan. I was terrified that the my medication would lead to some gross deformity in the baby. It was wonderful seeing all its bits in order. I can't decide whether to have a caesarean or a vaginal delivery and I still worry about the tiny chance that the baby will have HIV.

Everyone has been very supportive about the news.

This first appeared in the September 2004 edition of Positive Nation magazine.

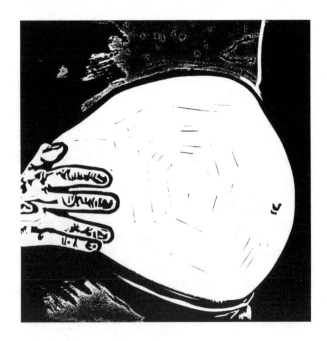

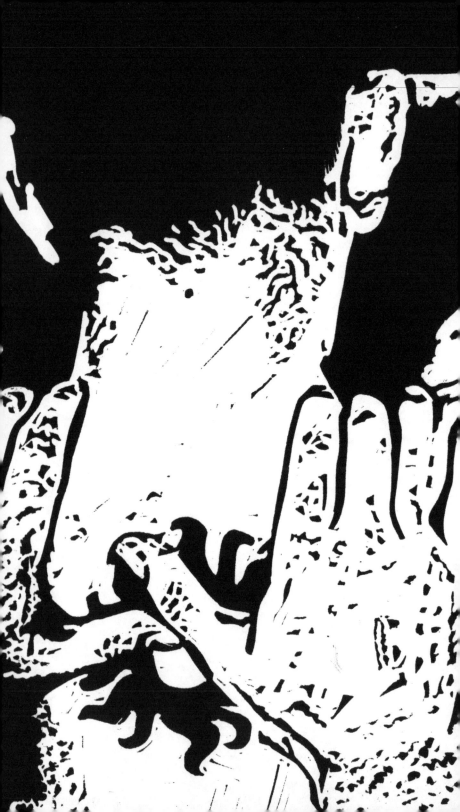

Complementary therapies

In this chapter you'll find information on

Why people use complementary therapies.

Some points to remember about complementary therapies and how to choose a therapist.

How to combine conventional and complementary therapies.

A list of complementary therapies.

There is a testimony from a man about how he looks after his health.

Reasons why people with HIV use complementary therapies

Complementary therapies are used by a large number of people with HIV.

There's no consensus amongst HIV doctors about the role of complementary therapies in the treatment of HIV. Some doctors dismiss them out of hand, whilst others take a more open-minded view. This is partly because complementary therapies have not, on the whole, been subjected to the same rigorous assessment of their effectiveness and safety as licensed medicines.

Reasons for the use of complementary therapies include stress reduction, the relief of side-effects and symptoms, to relieve pain, and to boost the immune system.

Reducing stress

Many people use complementary therapies to reduce stress. They can also have added benefits, such as increasing a general sense of health and well-being.

Reducing treatment side-effects

The side-effects of HIV treatment, and of the drugs used to treat infections, can be improved by supplements and complementary medicines. For example, calcium supplements can help control diarrhoea, a very common side-effect of HIV treatment. Aromatherapy oils, such as rosemary and peppermint, can relieve feelings of nausea; and herbs, such as valerian, and relaxation therapies can help with disturbed sleep and anxiety.

Boosting the immune system

There's very little evidence, partly due to a lack of research, that complementary therapies can boost the immune system, despite the fact that this benefit is claimed for many treatments.

Slowing HIV disease progression

It's known that people with HIV often have certain nutritional deficiencies. This is a symptom of HIV infection rather than a cause of immune deficiency or opportunistic infections. Providing supplementation may help address these deficiencies, but there's very limited evidence that this will lead to any improvement in immune function or health.

Pain relief

Some forms of complementary therapy can provide effective pain relief. Acupuncture is commonly used to relieve pain, and massage therapies and osteopathy can also be effective, particularly for muscle or joint pain. Always tell your doctor if you experience anything other than mild pain, or if you are in persistent pain.

Treatment for infections

There's no evidence that complementary medicines can prevent or cure any major infection. You will be endangering your life if you choose an alternative approach for the treatment of a major infection such as pneumonia, which always requires appropriate antibiotic treatment. Having said that, herbal remedies, acupuncture and homeopaths can help relieve some of the symptoms of infections, such as night sweats.

Points to remember

Complementary therapies will not solve your health or life problems, so be realistic in your expectations of what they can deliver. For example, question whether your chosen therapy will help control your symptoms or side-effects, or simply make them easier to live with.

Complementary treatments don't have the same methods of rigorous regulation and control as conventional medicine. For this reason, treat with suspicion the claims made about the effectiveness of any therapy you are considering.

Just like conventional medicine, complementary therapies can have side-effects or can even be dangerous. What's more, herbal remedies can interact with anti-HIV drugs. For example, the herbal treatment for depression, St John's wort, can reduce levels of protease inhibitors and NNRTIs in the blood. Large doses of vitamin C can lower blood concentrations of the protease inhibitor indinavir, and large doses of garlic have been shown to reduce the level of the protease inhibitor saquinavir. Just because a treatment is 'natural' doesn't mean that it's automatically safe or risk-free.

Choosing a therapist

Most complementary therapy practitioners will only see a few, if any, patients with HIV. It can therefore be hard to be confident that you are being treated by a practitioner who understands your situation. It's worth asking a few questions:

- What is the treatment you are offering and how can it benefit me? Different practitioners will approach the same therapy in different ways. If a practitioner makes amazing claims for the benefits of their therapy, such as an ability to cure HIV, they're best avoided, as is any practitioner who advises you to stop your anti-HIV treatment or other conventional treatment.

- What is your experience of treating people with HIV? It's important that your practitioner has a basic understanding of HIV. If they don't have this knowledge, they may miss important symptoms which you should bring to the attention of a doctor.

- What are your charges? Charges vary. Discuss and agree charges in advance. Be wary of any practitioner charging more than £60 for an initial assessment - the chances are that you're being overcharged. Many practitioners will have a sliding scale of fees depending on your income. Some HIV organisations offer some complementary therapies. These have been heavily cut back since effective anti-HIV treatments became available, so don't assume that a treatment you received for free in the past will still be available.

- What are your qualifications? Try and find out what qualification your practitioner has. This isn't necessarily a guarantee of competence or quality, as very few complementary therapies have the same rigorous regulation that governs conventional medicine.

Combining conventional and complementary therapies

Always tell your HIV doctor about any complementary therapies or supplements you may be using. Listen to any doubts your doctor might express about your chosen complementary approach. Although a good doctor will respect your choice, you should take note of any evidence he offers to show that a therapy doesn't have any benefit or is even harmful. On the other hand, if you have a major disagreement with your doctor it could be that another doctor at your HIV clinic has a more sympathetic attitude towards complementary therapies.

It's extremely important that you find out if you can combine your complementary therapies with your orthodox treatment. It's particularly important if you are taking herbal remedies or supplements of any kind. As mentioned before, some herbal remedies and supplements interact with anti-HIV drugs. As well as the interactions that are already known, there could well be others, as the way in which herbal remedies and medicines interact hasn't been studied very extensively.

You should tell your complementary therapist about any anti-HIV or other medicines you are receiving. This will help them to avoid interactions. Some complementary therapy practitioners take the view that orthodox medicines contribute to, or even cause, illness. They should, however, respect your choice to take conventional medicine.

It's always worth remembering that the dramatic improvements in the health of many people with HIV, and the fall in illness and deaths caused by HIV, are due to effective anti-HIV treatment. Treat with great suspicion any therapist who questions or denies this.

A-Z of complementary therapies

The following is a very brief introduction to some of the complementary and alternative therapies used by people with HIV. A lot more information can be found in NAM's Directory of complementary therapies in HIV and AIDS, which is available free to people affected by HIV.

Acupuncture

This is an aspect of traditional Chinese medicine (see entry below). It involves the insertion of fine needles into different points of the body to improve the flow of energy. This is normally painless or involves only very mild discomfort. It can be helpful with coping with stress, fatigue and pain.

Aromatherapy

This uses essential oils extracted from plants. Each oil is supposed to have a different healing effect on the mind and body. They can be directly inhaled, or used in baths or massage. Aromatherapy is an effective treatment for stress and encourages relaxation. Some oils can be toxic, so it's worth seeing a qualified aromatherapist.

Autogenic training

This is a technique using daily mental exercises to reduce stress, directing the mind and body towards a state of deep relaxation and encouraging healing. It is credited with increasing energy and helping with sleeping problems. It may also help with certain symptoms such as breathlessness or night sweats.

Bach flower remedies

These are harmless, inexpensive remedies available from many wholefood shops. They are derived from wild flowers and claim a wide range of calming and restorative powers.

Dietary therapies

Diet plays a key role in many complementary and alternative therapies, but there are certain diets which claim to improve health and immunity. These include macrobiotic diets, anti-candida diets and organic, raw and whole food diets. All may have advantages, but changing your whole diet at once can be very difficult, and if you are ill, or have metabolic complications, it might not be a good idea at all. See a dietitian before making any major changes to your diet (for more see the chapter *Nutrition and HIV*).

Exercise

Any form of vigorous exercise will help improve your cardiovascular fitness, reduce your risk of heart disease, help you to maintain lean muscle mass, and improve your ability to fight infection (see the chapter *Exercise*). Exercise such as T'ai chi, yoga and the Alexander technique are disciplines which many find calm the body, mind and spirit.

Healing and therapeutic touch

There are many forms of healing through touch, including some based on faith and therapies such as Reiki. All seek to encourage healing through one person acting as a channel for energy to flow into another. Reported results include improvements in mental or physical health and greater relaxation.

Herbs

This is a form of medicine which uses plants or herbs to maintain health, treat illness and promote health. Herbal treatments can be used successfully to treat minor ailments, such as tea tree oil or garlic for some fungal infections. However, bad reactions can occur and herbal treatments can interact with medicines used to treat HIV. Always tell your doctor about any herbal therapy you are taking or thinking of taking.

Homoeopathy

In homoeopathy, tiny traces of a substance that would normally cause illness are used to treat the same illness. Symptoms are not repressed but encouraged as they are seen as the body's way of healing itself, and homoeopathic remedies are finely tuned to each individual. Homoeopaths approach HIV in different ways. Some aim to treat a particular infection or illness, other will be more concerned with damage to the immune system. Homoeopaths are as likely to be interested in your emotional symptoms as your physical symptoms.

Hypnotherapy

The trance-like state created by a hypnotist opens the mind to suggestion, which can help reduce symptoms and help with psychological treatment. It can help reduce stress and pain. However, it's vital that you use a reputable practitioner.

Massage

This is one of the simplest and most popular therapies. It is an excellent way of reducing stress and promoting a sense of well-being and can help relieve some of the side-effects of anti-HIV treatment.

Naturopathy

This is a drug-free healing process based on the principle that the body is able to heal itself, supported by changes in diet, fasting, sweating and exercise. However, naturopaths acknowledge the importance of medicines when they are needed, and focus their therapy in this instance on improving overall health and well-being.

Osteopathy

This is a physical, manipulative therapy which seeks to correct any structural dysfunctions in the body that are causing health problems. Recurrent chest pain, neck pain, problems with swallowing, breathing and bowel function can all be improved with osteopathy. It's widely used for muscle and joint pain, and can also improve general vitality.

Reflexology

Reflexologists treat the bottom of your feet as a map for your body, and by massaging specific areas of the feet seek to improve the health of the related part of the body. Reflexology can offer relief for specific symptoms and side-effects as well as reducing stress.

Shiatsu

This is a combination of massage and acupuncture, where pressure is applied to healing points on the body, improving the flow of blood and energy and increasing vitality. It's an effective treatment for stress, anxiety and related conditions such as insomnia. It can also be used to treat symptoms and side-effects such as nausea.

Traditional Chinese medicine

This is a medical discipline which uses concepts, language and methods which are completely different from medicine practiced in the west. It incorporates several different elements including qi gong, acupuncture (see above) and herbal remedies. Qi gong and acupuncture both focus on the balance of the energies, 'qi', in the body. Chinese herbal medicine has been practiced for thousands of years, and works by strengthening the immune system rather than by directly attacking an infection. Chinese herbal medicine can cause side-effects, and can also interact with prescription medication.

Visualisation

This uses mental imagery to fight illness and has been credited with an improvement in symptoms and an increase in energy levels.

Further reading

- NAM factsheet, *Vitamins, minerals and herbal supplements.*

- *Anti-HIV drugs, HIV therapy* and *Nutrition* booklets in the information for HIV-positive people series produced by NAM.

- NAM's *Directory of Complementary Therapies in HIV and AIDS.*

- 'Drugs used by people with HIV' in NAM's *HIV and AIDS Treatments Directory.*

The Ikea approach

I've no doubt that the main reason that I'm alive and well after 15 years of living with HIV is because combination therapy became available in 1996, just as my immune system was starting to become so weak that I was vulnerable to AIDS-defining illnesses.

Well, eight years on, my CD4-cell count is over 1,000 and my viral load has been undetectable for years.

But as well as acknowledging how important HIV drugs have been, I also want to claim a bit of the credit for doing my bit to keep myself healthy and fit. It's what I call my "Ikea approach" (after the low-cost Swedish home furnishing store that keeps prices down by asking customers to collect their purchases from the warehouse, and assemble them themselves). Well, I met the medicines half-way by making sure I looked after myself.

First of all I make sure I take my anti-HIV pills. Okay, I've missed the odd dose, and taken some a few hours late. But I seem to have got away with it and am still taking my first combination (except for one change due to side-effects).

Then there's my diet. For the first few years after my HIV diagnosis I was obsessive about my diet, making sure that my diet, from my bowl of wholemeal porridge for breakfast, to my fruit salad desert after supper, was as healthy as possible. It may have been healthy, but it was also very worthy and, actually, boring. I'm now much more relaxed and more or less eat what I want, particularly as I once heard an HIV doctor say that being HIV-positive means "eating for two". Okay, I still make sure that I eat lots of fresh fruit and veg, and am easy on the lard, but now I allow myself food that I want to eat, not food that I feel I should eat.

I've always been pretty active and do a lot of exercise. Being honest, vanity was my main motivation to start off with - I found it was much easier to pull with a few muscles - but over the years, fitness and health has become more of a priority. I do a blend of weights and cardio and hope that's helped control my blood fats even though I'm taking a protease inhibitor.

At times I've used complementary and alternative treatments. For a few years, in the early 90s, I was actually quite into them. There seemed to be so little else I could do to fight HIV. I tried a few things, including acupuncture, high dose vitamins and Chinese herbs. Well, my T-cell count didn't go down when I was using them, but they still didn't prevent me getting a bad chest infection which meant a lengthy stay in hospital.

I do still use them though, but am realistic about what they can achieve. As far as I'm concerned, anti-HIV drugs are the reason I'm alive and well, the complementary stuff is just that - a desirable add-on, to help me feel more comfortable. Acupuncture helps me relax, and really did help to relieve the side-effects I experienced when I started my first combination. The odd massage makes me feel better, and I still take a multivitamin every morning. I figure it can't do me any harm, and might actually do me some good.

Having got my life back, I want to enjoy it. That hasn't always been easy. I've gone through some really bleak periods during the time I've had HIV and actually felt suicidal at times. Counselling helped at times, but at others talking about feeling bad and why I felt awful actually made things worse! Antidepressants helped a lot, though, as did some focused psychotherapy when I wasn't actually depressed.

Since I was a student, I've enjoyed a drink, and still do. I've also had some great times on drugs of various descriptions. Projectile vomiting and convulsing in a club after taking a pill a few months after starting HIV medicines was a bit of a wake-up call and I haven't touched anything since. I know a lot of people manage to mix medicines and recreationals, but that was just too frightening for me.

Just after my HIV diagnosis I bought a sofa from Ikea, thinking that as I wasn't going to last too long, it didn't matter if it didn't either. Well, the sofa, like me, is still here.

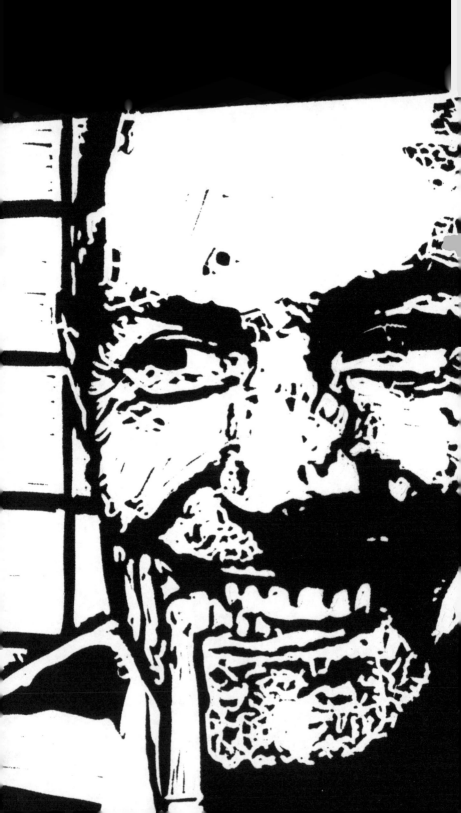

Daily health issues

In this chapter you'll find information on

Daily hygiene issues you may need to
think about.

Issues regarding pets, drinking water, food
safety, travel, vaccinations and sex.

Recreational drug use and safer drug use.

Day-to-day hygiene

Generally, hygiene precautions for people with HIV need not be different from those for anyone else. This is because most of the opportunistic infections associated with HIV are not ones you `catch' from the environment. For instance, people with HIV are no more or less vulnerable to the common cold than anyone else.

A few simple basic hygiene guidelines make good sense:

- Wash your hands thoroughly with soap and hot running water after using the toilet, handling rubbish or pet waste, and before and after preparing food.

- Wear strong rubber gloves and use very hot water and strong disinfectants when cleaning up anything messy such as diarrhoea, pet droppings and manure, or when gardening or dealing with rubbish.

- Make sure you use different cleaning cloths for kitchen surfaces and floors and the bathroom.

- If you have cuts on your skin, wash well under running water, encourage a bit of bleeding to flush out any germs, clean the cut with antiseptic and put a waterproof plaster over it.

- Get medical attention if you have a deep cut.

- Do not share toothbrushes or razors.

- Carefully dispose of sharp objects.

There are some other circumstances where it is worth taking extra precautions. Avoid children with chicken pox if you have never been exposed to it before. It is caused by the herpes zoster virus, which may cause shingles in HIV-positive adults.

Pets and animals

Some doctors warn that diseases such as toxoplasmosis, which can have very serious health implications for people whose immune systems are damaged, could be acquired from cats, birds or dogs. Others would agree that though this is true in theory, in practice, if you have owned your pet for a while, there may be no extra risk to you. This is because of the nature of opportunistic infections. Most of them involve the activation or reactivation of micro-organisms which entered the body in the past. On that basis, if you have had a particular pet for a while, you are unlikely to be at risk of catching anything new from it.

There is also evidence to suggest that the risk of acquiring such infections from animals is, in reality, low. One study has reported that people with HIV who owned cats were no more likely to develop toxoplasmosis during their illness than those who did not own cats. Changing cat litter on a daily basis will reduce the risk of toxoplasmosis. Clean the litter tray using rubber gloves, hot water and strong disinfectants.

Cats can also harbour the bacterial infection *Bartonella* (also known as `cat scratch' disease). Try not to let your cat lick open cuts, and try to ensure that it doesn't get fleas, as all of these can transmit *Bartonella*. Always wash your hands between touching pets and handling food.

Exposure to potentially harmful organisms can also occur when working with animals or gardening. For example, cleaning chicken coops or cleaning up pigeon droppings could expose HIV-positive people to infections, as could gardening without gloves.

If your job could lead to you coming into contact with potentially dangerous infections, then you should discuss this with your doctor and the occupational health department at your work.

Drinking water

On the whole, it's safe for people with HIV to drink water from the tap in the UK.

But if you have a severely damaged immune system, a little more caution might be needed. Water companies cannot guarantee that water supplies are free from cryptosporidium or other similar organisms which cause diarrhoea in HIV-positive people who have very low CD4 cell counts. Once contracted, cryptosporidium seems impossible to eliminate in HIV-positive people who have CD4 counts below 200 and leads to serious diarrhoea and inability to absorb food or fluids. It is a serious opportunistic infection, against which current treatments are only partially successful.

People who have CD4 cell counts above 200 appear to have developed enough immune response to control cryptosporidiosis, although they may experience some diarrhoea.

There were several outbreaks of cryptosporidiosis in London and Oxfordshire in the early 1990s, which caused severe diarrhoea even in HIV-negative people. These outbreaks have been traced to the water supply.

Thames Water, which provides water in London, says that it is impossible to filter drinking water for the cryptosporidium egg because the infectious dose is so low. Hundreds of gallons of water would need to be screened to find one egg. Unlike bacterial infections, which are able to establish themselves only when tens of thousands of bacteria get into the gut, ten cryptosporidium eggs are enough to cause severe diarrhoea.

If you fit your own filter against cryptosporidium, it should have a very fine mesh.

Filtered water should be kept in the fridge. If it is left at room temperature, it may actually be more vulnerable to bacterial contamination than plain tap water because filtering removes the chlorine which is added to water supplies. The main drawback of filtered water is the cost; over £100 for the filter and fitting.

The only other way to eliminate the organism is to boil drinking water for at least one minute. Such a lengthy boiling period is necessary in order to ensure that all the water has reached boiling point; an automatic kettle switches off when the water in contact with the filament has reached boiling point. Some experts on water safety say that this is not long enough to ensure the elimination of some organisms.

Many people assume that bottled mineral water is always safe, but this is definitely not true. Bottled water sources cannot be screened for cryptosporidium either, and other bacteria not present in chlorinated tap water have been found in some brands of bottled water.

It is important to remember that drinking water includes the water with which you brush your teeth and prepare or wash food (for people with CD4 counts below 200, this means being careful all the time). Drinking water also includes ice in drinks, which is made from tap water.

Drinking water may also contain other diarrhoea-causing bacteria. These have been isolated in bottled water as well as tap water, and the only way to

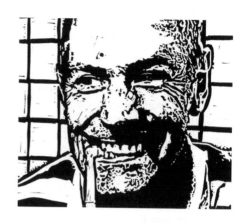

remove these bacteria is either to boil water or to use a very fine mesh filter, even finer than the filters recommended for cryptosporidium. Jug filters, which are very popular, tend to remove chemical impurities but may not always screen out bacteria.

To make life easier, it may help to boil up water once a day and keep it in the fridge to use later on. Don't use boiled water that is over twelve hours old, even if it has been kept in the fridge.

Unfortunately, it is not always possible to monitor the quality of water which you drink or which is used in the preparation of food outside the home. In these circumstances, the best policy may be to avoid salads and other raw foods, and to drink bottled water from deep mountain springs, which are least likely to be contaminated with cryptosporidium.

Beer, pasteurised fruit juice and bottled/canned soft drinks do not carry the risk of cryptosporidium infection, but it's unknown whether wine could carry the infection.

Water outside the UK can present problems. Even in other European countries it is best to stick to boiled water or, if this is difficult, bottled water that comes from deep mountain springs. In tropical and subtropical countries, water presents a very serious health hazard to HIV-positive people. A large number of gut infections are water-borne, including some which cause life-threatening diarrhoea, and any traveller who returns from these countries with diarrhoea will tell you that, however tempting it may look, roadside food and drink is not worth the risk.

Swimming in the sea or in rivers may also be inadvisable for people with compromised immune systems, especially off the British coast. Several recent reports have highlighted extensive problems with water-borne infections contracted from polluted or sewage-ridden water. This is also known to be a problem in many Mediterranean resorts and a cautious approach would be to swim only in chlorinated swimming pools.

Food poisoning

If you have a strong immune system, your risk of getting food poisoning is no greater than it is for an HIV-negative person.

However, food poisoning can be a lot more severe in people with AIDS. It makes sense for everyone who has a low CD4 count to take extra precautions.

Salmonella is a definite risk for people with HIV. Salmonella is as much a problem in Britain as it is in other parts of the world. Another possible risk is listeria, another infection spread by food, which may cause particular problems for children with HIV. Shigella and campylobacter can also cause problems. Infections with these organisms can be hard to get rid of, and they can fail to respond to treatments which are effective in HIV-negative people.

Salmonella frequently infects chickens. This means that it is especially important to make sure chicken is cooked through, so that no red blood can be seen at all. Take special care with frozen chicken. Meat should be thawed in the fridge, not at room temperature. Wash your hands after handling uncooked poultry and make sure uncooked meat and poultry is not stored uncovered in the fridge near cold meats or dairy products. Ideally, wash eggs before cracking them, and cook them thoroughly until both the yolk and the white set. Do not use cracked eggs.

It is also advisable to avoid unpasteurised dairy products, including unpasteurised milk, 'live' yoghurt and some soft cheeses, which may also contain salmonella and listeria. Some people have advocated live yoghurt as a treatment for thrush. Although there is some evidence that this does indeed have benefits, it is important that people with HIV are aware that it may also carry some risk.

It may also be sensible to avoid farm animals and their droppings, since these can harbour infections such as cryptosporidium. Organically grown vegetables are often grown in a medium that includes raw manure, so it is wise to brush off as much dirt as possible and then clean the vegetables with boiled water.

If reheating or microwaving food, take care to ensure that it is properly cooked all the way through. Wash fruit and vegetables properly, and keep cutting and preparation surfaces clean. When on holiday in warm climates, the risk of food poisoning may well extend to salads and fruit. Food which you know has been immediately and thoroughly cooked is safest. Do not use food after its sell-by date.

International travel

Going to a foreign country can be daunting, as even straightforward everyday tasks may suddenly require learning a whole new set of steps. Just the strain of daily life can become stressful. In addition, you are likely to be exposed to new and potentially dangerous bugs for which your immune system will be unprepared. It is wise to have a check-up at your clinic before you go, and to ask about any extra precautions you need to take. If you are currently using any medications, ensure that you take an adequate supply with you, as they may be hard or impossible to obtain abroad. Medicines should be clearly labelled, and, at some countries' customs and immigration points, it will help to have a doctor's letter stating that you need the treatments. There's a lot more information on travelling with your medication in the chapter *Travel*.

It is sensible to research local medical facilities before travelling to another country, particularly if local medical care is likely to be relatively poor.

Make sure that you have the right travel and medical insurance. Most policies won't cover medical conditions that you know were aware of when you took out the policy. For more on travel insurance, see the chapter *Travel*.

Coughs are a common problem among travellers, and you may be at particular risk during air travel, when large numbers of people are confined in a small space, breathing recirculated air.

Travellers' diarrhoea is usually caused by the contamination of food or water with faecal bacteria by people who have not washed their hands. It affects about 40% of travellers to developing countries, even when they have perfectly intact immune systems, and can be a particular problem for people with HIV. The most common cause of diarrhoea after travelling is giardiasis, which can be treated quite easily in people with HIV.

Vaccinations and immunisations

An immunisation (often called a vaccination) is designed to protect the recipient against an infectious disease. People with HIV should receive the vaccinations against hepatitis A virus and hepatitis B virus. It's not recommended that people with HIV receive live vaccines such as the BCG tuberculosis jab, as this might cause illness.

Sex

There are good reasons why you should still consider having safer sex even if you are HIV-positive.

First of all, you might infect somebody else with HIV. In England, there have been cases of men being sent to prison for infecting their sexual partners with HIV, and a man has also been imprisoned in Scotland for this.

Then there's the issue of sexually transmitted infections, which at the very least can be unpleasant and inconvenient, and can also make it more likely that you can pass on HIV during sex. If left untreated, some sexually transmitted infections can cause serious health problems, particularly if your immune system is very weak.

There is some evidence that unsafe sex might damage the health of people with HIV and several cases of reinfection or superinfection with drug-resistant strains of HIV have now been presented.

In the early 1990s, an American study involving thousands of HIV-positive gay men found that men who had unprotected anal sex experienced faster disease progression and became ill with HIV-related illnesses faster than those who said they only had safer sex. A study involving Kenyan sex workers showed that women who had unprotected sex had more sexually transmitted infections and lower CD4 cell counts.

For more information see the chapter *Sex and HIV*.

Reinfection/superinfection

Although it is clearly established that drug-resistant HIV can be transmitted to previously uninfected people, it is less clear if it can be transmitted to people already infected with HIV. There have, however, been several case reports from around the world of HIV-positive people being reinfected with another strain of HIV after having unprotected sex - and doing less well on their HIV treatment as a consequence.

It seems that reinfection is, however, rare, and in a number of the reported cases the individuals were taking a break from their HIV treatment when they became reinfected

This is quite a controversial subject. It is being looked at very closely by doctors around the world, and more information is being published on it all the time.

Different strains of HIV

Many different strains of HIV exist, some of which are more aggressive than others in the test-tube. It has been suggested that transmission of an aggressive strain (to an individual who is already infected with a less aggressive strain) may trigger the onset of AIDS.

This might happen because the aggressive strain could overwhelm the immune system. For instance, a person's immune system may have responded quite successfully to initial HIV infection, so that the dominant strain of HIV in the body is one which is less harmful to the host. Reinfection with another strain could tip this balance: the host's immune system may be unable to contain a new, more aggressive virus strain, which could therefore be able to replicate rapidly. The aggressive new virus could soon overtake the strain already present, and become the dominant strain. Another theory is that the new strains might selectively infect certain types of cells or tissues which had been largely unaffected previously, and so lead to faster disease progression.

It has certainly been demonstrated that people have been infected with two different subtypes of HIV, but no one is sure when those infections might have occurred. Some researchers have suggested that infection with a second strain of HIV is most likely to occur in the first few months of primary infection, because this is the time when the immune response against HIV is least strong. Others argue that the immune response may not be protective, and that re-infection could occur at a later stage.

Co-factors
Although there are these doubts about the importance of re-infection with HIV, there are reasons to believe that other virus infections and sexually transmitted infections may speed up disease progression.

In the first place, many infections are likely to cause HIV to reproduce simply because they stimulate the immune system. That immune response will include the activation of latent HIV in immune cells, leading to the production of new HIV and the infection of further cells.

For instance, after being infected with cytomegalovirus (CMV), people with HIV infection have been shown to suffer increases in HIV replication. But CMV and some other viruses can also assist HIV in the infection of new cells, and speed up HIV replication in cells which are infected with both HIV and CMV. The same goes for other herpes viruses, Epstein-Barr virus (which causes glandular fever) and hepatitis B virus. All these viruses have the potential to provide 'keys' to cells which HIV would otherwise be unable to infect. Almost all of these viruses are transmitted through sexual or body fluid contact.

Sexually transmitted infections
For most people with HIV, standard treatments for sexually transmitted infections work just as well as they do in HIV-negative people.

However, if your immune system is very weak, you might need a longer course of antibiotics to treat infections such as gonorrhoea and syphilis.

Viral sexually transmitted infections can also be more serious and harder to treat if you have HIV. For example, people with HIV may be at greater risk of having more frequent and more painful attacks of genital herpes.

In people with HIV, it can also be harder for the immune system to clear infection with HPV, the virus that causes genital and anal warts. Some strains of this virus can cause cervical and anal cancer, and even after the introduction of anti-HIV treatments, doctors have seen an increase in the incidence of these cancers in people with HIV.

Hepatitis B virus is also sexually transmittable, and people with HIV are recommended to be vaccinated against it. There's evidence that hepatitis C virus can also be sexually transmitted.

Oral-anal contact, or rimming, can lead to gut infections.

It is up to each individual to decide what sex practices they want to keep up, which they want to modify, and which they want to stop. For instance, one might still make the choice not to use condoms for penetrative sex with a regular HIV-positive partner. At the other end of the spectrum, one might decide to begin to use condoms for oral sex.

Recreational drug use

Nearly every person with HIV uses some form of drug. Most people use legal drugs like coffee, tea or chocolate, and many others drink alcohol or smoke tobacco. A large number of people with HIV also use illegal drugs.

In this section, information is provided on alcohol, tobacco and so-called recreational drugs.

Drugs and the law

For the very latest information on the adverse effects and legal status of drugs, you might want to look at the website of the UK drugs information charity Drugscope, www.drugscope.org.uk.

Generally, drugs in the UK are controlled by two laws: the Medicines Act and the Misuse of Drugs Act. The Medicines Act bans the non-medical use of some licensed pharmaceuticals. The Misuse of Drugs Act is concerned with the use of banned drugs, which are placed into different categories. Offences involving Class A drugs carry the stiffest penalties, and offences involving Class C drugs the lightest. A first offence involving possession of drugs is likely to involve a fine or caution. But this would mean that you have a criminal record. Regular offenders, and people who sell or smuggle drugs, can expect to face a prison sentence, and having HIV is unlikely to mean that the courts will deal with you more leniently.

Alcohol

Alcohol is a drug and comes in many forms, including beer, cider, wine, 'alcopops' and spirits such as whisky, gin and vodka.

Alcohol is legally available in the UK from licensed outlets to people aged over 18 years and is enjoyed and used safely by many people. However, alcohol is a major cause of health and social problems, and, after tobacco, causes more deaths in the UK than any other drug.

Alcohol relaxes the brain and body, and is normally drunk for its pleasant effects. Because of its power to alter mood and make physical changes, it can also lead to physical, psychological and social problems. Many people find that moderate drinking (a unit or two of alcohol per day) helps relieve stress, encourages relaxation and acts as an appetite stimulant. A unit of alcohol is equal to a half-pint of normal strength beer or lager, a pub measure of spirits, a glass of wine, or a small glass of sherry or port.

Health agencies recommend that men should not drink more than 3 to 4 units of alcohol per day. For women, the daily limit is 2 to 3 units. This advice applies regardless of whether you drink daily, weekly or somewhere in between. Drinking all your weekly limit in one session (often called binge drinking) can lead to poor coordination, vomiting, exaggerated emotional reactions (including sadness, tearfulness, anger and aggression) and can even cause unconsciousness. Women who are pregnant, or planning to become so, are advised to drink no more than 1 to 2 units per week.

A hangover the next day - headache, dry mouth, feeling sick and tired - is a very common consequence of heavy drinking the night before. These effects are caused by dehydration and toxicities, so if you drink alcohol, you should drink plenty of water as well.

As even small amounts of alcohol can have an effect on your coordination, reactions and judgments, you should never drink even small amounts of alcohol and then drive or operate machinery.

Extremely heavy drinking can lead to coma and even death.

Long-term heavy alcohol consumption (10 or more units a day in a man or 6 or more in a woman) can cause ill health, affecting the liver, heart and brain. Drinking every day can also lead to physical and psychological dependence on alcohol.

In addition, people who drink heavily often don't eat well and this can cause further health problems. Alcohol is a depressive drug and can cause or make worse mental, psychological or emotional problems. Used in conjunction with other drugs, such as over-the-counter painkillers like paracetamol, alcohol can have more serious effects.

There is no evidence that moderate drinking (a unit or two of alcohol a day) does any harm to people with HIV. However, if you have hepatitis or high levels of blood fats, then you may have to cut down your alcohol consumption or stop drinking alcohol altogether.

Heavy drinking can affect your immune system and may slow down recovery from infections.

Heavy alcohol use can have potentially serious consequences for people taking anti-HIV drugs. Alcohol is processed by the liver and a healthy liver is necessary for the body to process medicines effectively. The blood fat increases caused by some anti-HIV drugs can be made worse by heavy drinking.

People who have hepatitis as well as HIV are advised not to drink alcohol at all, or to keep alcohol consumption to an absolute minimum.

People whose liver has been damaged by drinking too much alcohol (especially if they have hepatitis) are more likely to experience side-effects from anti-HIV drugs, particularly protease inhibitors.

Alcohol can react badly with certain medicines (for example some anti-TB drugs and some antibiotics) so it is a good idea to check with your pharmacist whether it is safe to drink alcohol with any new medicines you may be prescribed. However, there is no significant interaction between any of the currently available anti-HIV drugs and alcohol.

Alcohol can cause vomiting. If you vomit within an hour of taking a dose of your anti-HIV drugs, or any other medicine you have been told to take, you should retake the dose.

If you are concerned about your drinking, speak to a member of your healthcare team, who will be able to direct you to somebody who can help. Alcohol Concern, one of the UK's largest alcohol charities, can be contacted via www.alcoholconcern.org.uk, or phone Drinkline on 0800 917 8282. More information on Scottish support services is online at www.alcohol-focus-scotland.org.uk, or phone 0141 576 6700.

Amphetamines (speed)
Also see the section on crystal meth below

Amphetamines are stimulants normally taken orally, although they can be dissolved in water, snorted, or injected. After cannabis, amphetamines are the most widely used illicit drug in the UK, and are classified as a Class B drug in the Misuse of Drugs Act, unless they are prepared for injection, when they are Class A.

Amphetamines cause the heart rate to increase, appetite to diminish, mood to improve, and the pupils to dilate. Users often report a 'rush' of confidence lasting three or four hours before they begin to 'come down'. Feelings of anxiety and agitation take over from this point. Repeated use of amphetamines can lead to tolerance of the drug, meaning that you have to take more to achieve a 'high'. Symptoms of anxiety, paranoia and panic can also set in. Prolonged and heavy use can lead to mental disturbances.

Amphetamine use postpones, but does not remove, the need to eat. Regular users often suffer from weight loss and malnutrition. This reduces the body's ability to fight infection, and this is a major concern for people with HIV.

There is no clear evidence that HIV-positive users of amphetamine experience faster disease progression, but see the section on crystal meth (methamphetamine).

Anabolic steroids
Anabolic steroids are hormones which are commonly used as drugs to build muscle mass. Body builders and, increasingly, regular gym users often use anabolic steroids in four-week cycles, to improve the effects of their training.

HIV-positive men are sometimes prescribed anabolic steroids or testosterone replacement therapy if they have low natural levels of testosterone or have lost a lot of lean muscle mass.

Steroids can be highly toxic to the liver, and can also cause acne, male pattern baldness, sexual problems and shrinking of the testicles. Women who use anabolic steroids can develop masculine characteristics.

Steroids bought at gyms are often counterfeit or contaminated in some way and can be particularly toxic to the liver and cause nerve damage.

There is controversy about the effect of anabolic steroids on the immune system. Some researchers have argued that they are immunosuppressive, but a study looking at the immune systems of HIV-positive men given prescribed steroid treatment for wasting showed that they did not suppress the immune system. However, it is known that steroid use can increase levels of LDL (bad) cholesterol, so they should be used with extreme caution and under close medical supervision if you have raised blood fats due to your anti-HIV medication.

Needle-sharing by steroid users carries exactly the same risk of HIV transmission as needle-sharing for recreational drug use.

Barbiturates (downers)

Barbiturates are used medically, to calm people down and as sleeping pills. Barbiturates are a prescription-only drug and are classified as a Class B drug if they are used illicitly. Possession is not, however, a criminal offence.

Barbiturates affect the central nervous system, causing a clammy feeling, and depending on the dose, the effects last between three and six hours. They can cause clumsiness, happiness and mental confusion - and unhappiness can also be caused by barbiturates.

Large doses can cause unconsciousness, breathing problems and death. Death from overdose is a very real danger, as there is a fine line between a safe and a dangerous dose. The chances of overdose are increased if barbiturates are taken with alcohol. The risks of barbiturate use are increased if the drug is injected.

The body can rapidly become tolerant of barbiturates, leading to both physical and mental dependence. Withdrawal can involve symptoms of irritability, sleeplessness, sickness, twitching, convulsions and delirium.

Heavy users are more vulnerable to chest complaints and hypothermia.

Cannabis

The legal status of cannabis changed recently in the UK, when the drug was reclassified from Class B to Class C.

Cannabis can be smoked, usually with tobacco, eaten, drunk in a 'tea' or snorted as a snuff. The drug affects the central nervous system and, as a result, users may experience relief from pain, feel light-headed, relaxed or sleepy. The drug can also stimulate appetite; the so-called 'munchies'. However, cannabis is also known to impair co-ordination, and can cause nausea and vomiting as well as anxiety and paranoia, which, with long-term use, may become chronic.

Medicinal use of cannabis is illegal and therefore there is little verifiable evidence of the drug's effects when used in the management of chronic health conditions. However, cannabis is widely used illegally for medicinal reasons, often for the relief of pain or as an appetite stimulant. In 1996, a clinical trial in San Francisco found that people with HIV wasting disease who used cannabis were more likely to put on weight. The drug is also widely used to relieve insomnia and the symptoms of anxiety and stress. It is also used by people with multiple sclerosis as a muscle relaxant.

In recent years a small number of people have been prosecuted for growing and consuming cannabis for medical purposes. In most cases a suspended sentence has been issued, but recently a jury returned a not guilty verdict, and in another example a judge threw out the case.

The UK Government is currently reviewing the evidence on cannabis use. Cannabis extracts, called cannabinoids, are already legally used in licensed pharmaceuticals, mostly painkillers and muscle relaxants, but these can only be obtained on prescription. These products do not make users feel 'high' or have any of the other narcotic effects of cannabis.

Short-term risks of cannabis use include anxiety, panic, and paranoia. Memory and attention may also be affected, as might the ability to drive or operate machinery. Research suggests that cannabis use in teenagers is a predictor of later mental health problems. Use during pregnancy has been associated with low birth-weight babies.

If the drug is smoked, long-term use is known to cause many smoking-related respiratory and cardiovascular diseases such as asthma, bronchitis, emphysema and heart disease. This may be of particular concern to people with HIV who have suffered lung damage from TB, or to those with increased lipids from anti-HIV medication, as this may increase the risk of heart attack. There is also evidence that smoking cannabis can cause cancers of the mouth, throat and lungs.

Chronic loss of memory and shortened attention span have been observed in long-term users of the drug, in some cases even after their use has ceased, and there is evidence that long-term users can develop psychological dependency on the drug. In a recent survey, daily use of cannabis by teenagers was found to substantially increase the risk of developing depression later in life and the use of cannabis has also been linked with an increased risk of schizophrenia.

It is not known how cannabis reacts with anti-HIV drugs. A small American study found that cannabis use did not impact on the effectiveness of the protease inhibitor indinavir (*Crixivan*), even though the drugs use the same mechanism to pass through the body. Like any mood- or consciousness-altering drug, cannabis may have an impact on people's ability to adhere to their medication schedule. People planning to use cannabis, or any other recreational drug, may need to develop strategies to help them take their medication at the right time and in the right way.

Cocaine

Along with most other recreational drugs, government statistics suggest that more people are using cocaine (coke, charlie, snow, powder, marching powder) and the cocaine derivative, crack (freebase). In the UK, both cocaine and crack are illegal class A drugs. Dealing carries a maximum penalty of life imprisonment and unlimited fine, and possession can mean up to seven years in prison and a large fine.

Cocaine is a stimulant made from the leaves of the South American coca shrub. It comes in the form of a white powder, costing between £30 and £100 per gram. Usually snorted into the nose, it provides a feeling of excitement, exhilaration and self-confidence lasting for about 15-30 minutes. Cocaine can also be rubbed into the gums and into the anus or vagina before penetrative sex. Rarely, cocaine is also made into a solution for injection.

Crack is sold in the form of small rocks, which are smoked either in cigarettes or in a pipe. Historically, crack has been associated with poor urban populations, but is in fact used by people from a wide social spectrum.

Cocaine users may take many doses to maintain the high, which can cause anxiety, paranoia and a tolerance for the drug, meaning that larger doses have to be taken to achieve a similar high. Although not addictive in the same way as heroin or opiates, users can become psychologically dependent on the transient high which cocaine provides and find that they suffer anxiety, depression or severe tiredness if they stop using the drug.

Longer-term use of both cocaine and crack can cause severe anxiety, clinical depression, psychotic episodes, aggression, weight loss and malnutrition. Both drugs have also been shown to cause potentially fatal heart problems including heart attack, angina, irregular heart beat and inflammation and enlargement of the heart.

In common with most other street drugs, users are rarely sold a pure form of cocaine. The drug is often 'cut' with other cheaper drugs such as amphetamines (speed), talc or detergents, which can be poisonous or cause irritation, leading to infection.

Snorting cocaine can damage the membrane between the nostrils, leading to bleeding and eventual erosion. There have been reports that sharing snorting equipment may permit the transmission of hepatitis C virus. Rubbing cocaine into the gums, vagina, or anus can cause ulceration, which could increase transmission of HIV or other sexually transmitted infections. Sharing injecting equipment also presents a risk for transmission of HIV, hepatitis viruses and other blood-borne infections.

Cocaine is not metabolised by the body in the same way as anti-HIV drugs, so there does not appear to be cause for concern about interactions between them.

Test-tube studies suggest that cocaine alters the functioning of the immune system in several ways, making immune cells more vulnerable to HIV. Experiments conducted in HIV-infected mice bred in laboratories found that mice exposed to cocaine had far fewer CD4 cells than mice not given the drug. This suggests that HIV disease may progress faster in regular cocaine users.

However, studies looking at regular cocaine use and disease progression in gay men have produced conflicting results. One study found no association, whilst another found that weekly cocaine use was associated with a greater risk of death. Because drug use may be an indicator of other social issues which may have a negative effect on health - such as poor access to health care, or other health problems - these types of studies can be difficult to interpret.

As with all recreational drugs, it is also wise to consider how use could impact on adherence to your HIV treatments. If you are worried about your recreational drug use, then your doctor or health care team will be able to refer you to an appropriate source of support.

Crystal meth (methamphetamine)

Also know as crystal meth, ice, tina, krank, or yaba, methamphetamine is a synthetic form of amphetamine, a stimulant drug.

Crystal meth has been popular on the US gay scene for over a decade, and there have been some alarmist reports about its use amongst gay men in the UK and Europe. However, it is unclear just how widespread use of the drug, which is very expensive and difficult to obtain, actually is.

Methamphetamine is a class A drug.

Methamphetamine can be bought as a pill, as powder to be snorted through the nose or injected, or in a crystal form - ice - which is smoked in a pipe.

Methamphetamine brings on a rapid feeling of exhilaration, a perceived sharpening of focus and heightened sexual desire.

Smoking crystals of methamphetamine causes a rise in body temperature, an increased heart rate and rapid breathing.

Paranoia, short-term memory loss, rages and mood swings have been recorded.

There is anecdotal evidence that use of methamphetamine can cause people to become ill because of HIV more rapidly, to take more time to recover from infections and to respond less well to anti-HIV treatments. However, some people believe that this has a lot to do with users of the drug not taking their anti-HIV and other medication properly.

Rapid fall in CD4 cell count has been observed in methamphetamine users. However, as many users of methamphetamine have difficulty sleeping or eating properly, there may be other lifestyle factors involved in the quicker disease progression noted in some users.

Psychological dependence on the drug has also been reported, although it does not seem to cause physical addiction.

Taking large amounts of the drug can cause convulsions, problems with blood circulation, inability to breath, coma and death. However, deaths have been reported in people who have taken only small doses.

In the US there have been concerns about a link between the use of methamphetamine by gay men and unprotected sex, particularly when used in conjunction with drugs to treat erectile dysfunction, such as *Viagra* and *Cialis*.

There has been a case report of an interaction between methamphetamine and the protease inhibitor ritonavir (*Norvir*). Methamphetamine is metabolised by the body using the same mechanism as ritonavir. Doctors also believe that inhaling poppers may make the interaction worse.

The use of any drug can interfere with normal sleeping patterns, affect appetite and interrupt routines. Some people have found that this is particularly the case with methamphetamine. If you are using the drug, it makes sense to consider how it might affect issues such as adherence to your anti-HIV medication. The drug has also been linked with an increased likelihood of having unprotected sex, so plan how to manage this.

Ecstasy

Ecstasy (E, X) is an illegal class A drug. Dealing carries a maximum life prison sentence and unlimited fine, and possession up to seven years in prison and a £5,000 fine.

Ecstasy has both stimulant and hallucinogenic properties. Its active ingredient is a synthetic drug called MDMA. Originally used in psychotherapy, from the late 1970s it started to be used on the club scene due to its ability to reduce inhibitions, give an energy boost, induce relaxation and give intense pleasure by releasing the neurotransmitter serotonin.

The drug is sold in tablet form and, less frequently, as a powder. After about 30 to 45 minutes, the drug gives an intense 'high', which may last for several hours. Because the body becomes tolerant of the drug, people may end up taking larger quantities to induce similar feelings of euphoria.

Because ecstasy is illegal there have been no proper clinical trials looking at the risks of using the drug for people with HIV. The effects of ecstasy on the immune system and on HIV disease progression are therefore uncertain.

In 1996, a man who had recently started taking a combination of anti-HIV drugs, including the protease inhibitor ritonavir (*Norvir*), died after taking two and a half ecstasy tablets. An autopsy found that there was an unusually high amount of ecstasy in his blood, which may be partly explained by an interaction between the drug and ritonavir. Ritonavir boosts the amount of ecstasy in the bloodstream by between 200% and 300%, because the body uses the same process to break down both ritonavir and ecstasy.

Because other protease inhibitors (and NNRTIs and many other drugs) are metabolised using a similar process, there is a risk that ecstasy could interact dangerously with them, and there have been hospitalisations due to adverse reactions to ecstasy amongst people taking protease inhibitors.

If you've started a new treatment combination recently, the first four weeks, when your body gets used to the new drugs, are likely to be the riskiest time for interactions. Some doctors suggest that after this period, if you choose to take ecstasy, it may be safer to begin with a quarter or half a tablet first. This information is included here in order to help readers reduce risks, and has not been researched scientifically.

As with all recreational drugs, it is difficult to know what the ecstasy tablet you are using really contains. The doses found in street drugs are not controlled, and the ecstasy pill you buy might contain much larger quantities of the drug. Often, ecstasy will have been 'cut' with other substances which could be poisonous, or with other drugs, usually amphetamines or LSD, but occasionally heroin.

In the short term, ecstasy can cause dehydration, headache, chills, eye twitching, jaw clenching, blurred vision, nausea and vomiting and, like many drugs taken to get 'high', is commonly accompanied by a 'come-down'.

People can have an allergic reaction to the drug, which can be fatal (though deaths related to ecstasy are very rare in comparison to the extent of its consumption). The drug has also been associated with heart and lung problems, dramatic increases in body temperature, kidney failure and liver damage. The potential liver toxicities of ecstasy and other recreational drugs are of particular concern to people with HIV, as liver damage can itself make you very ill as well as stopping the body from processing anti-HIV drugs properly.

Long-term use has been linked to poor mental health, depression, psychotic episodes and memory problems.

If you are using ecstasy or planning to do so, then think about discussing this with your doctor or another member of your health care team. Most are quite happy to discuss drug use and can provide helpful information on minimising risks.

As with all recreational drugs, it is wise to consider how use could impact on adherence to your HIV treatments or other areas of your health or life.

GHB

GHB (gammahydroxybutyrate) has recently become popular on the club scene, with users reporting an alcohol-like high with potent positive sexual effects. However, its possession and use recently became illegal after a series of deaths were associated with its use.

GHB affects the release of dopamine in the brain, causing effects ranging from relaxation to deep sleep, and coma. The drug also lowers blood pressure and can cause breathing difficulties.

A case has been reported in which levels of GHB were increased to life-threatening levels when taken along with a protease inhibitor. A man who was taking ritonavir and saquinavir became deeply unconscious after taking a half-teaspoon of GHB. Doctors believe that the ritonavir and saquinavir slowed down the metabolism of GHB and caused a near-fatal reaction.

Heroin
See opiates

Ketamine
Ketamine is an anaesthetic which makes people feel detached from their immediate environment.

Since early 2006 possession of ketamine has been a crime. It comes in a white powder which can be snorted, dissolved or injected. It normally takes effect after about 20 minutes. The body heats up and users have reported a range of different experiences including an altered sense of their body, hallucinations, difficulty moving or even completely freezing. This is often called a 'K-hole', and involves difficulty communicating and even breathing and swallowing.

The effects of long-term ketamine use include memory loss and psychological disturbance. Several deaths have been reported due to the use of the drug in the UK. Although no specific interactions with anti-HIV medication have been reported, use of the drug could affect adherence to anti-HIV medication.

LSD

LSD (lysergic acid diethylamide, often known as acid) is a Class A drug. It is taken orally and normally begins to take effect after about 30 to 60 minutes. Its hallucinogenic effects last up to eight hours, although some people report "trips" lasting as long as 24 hours.

LSD is not thought to affect the immune system and no specific interactions with anti-HIV drugs have been reported. However, when 'tripping' on acid adherence to anti-HIV medication might be difficult or even impossible.

Opiates

These include heroin and methadone and are made from the opium poppy. Heroin is a Class A drug. Methadone is controlled by the Medicines Act.

Opiates are normally injected, smoked or sniffed. They depress the nervous system and have a euphoric effect. Tolerance of opiates develops quickly, as does dependence.

Use of opiates can cause chest problems and constipation. Sharing the equipment used to inject opiates can lead to infection with tetanus, hepatitis B and C, HIV, and can cause blood poisoning and abscesses.

Use of opiates can lead to malnutrition and self-neglect.

Methadone is a form of opiate normally supplied on prescription to registered addicts as an alternative to injecting. It is usually taken as a liquid. To withdraw from opiate use, addicts can gradually reduce their dose of methadone over a long period of time.

Methadone interacts with anti-HIV drugs. The drug is known to increase levels of AZT (zidovudine, *Retrovir*) in the blood. Doctors are often very cautious about giving protease inhibitors to people taking methadone, and will often admit them to hospital for observation for a short time. The protease inhibitor nelfinavir (*Viracept*) reduces methadone levels. The NNRTIs have differing effects on methadone levels. Nevirapine (*Viramune*) increases levels of methadone, whereas efavirenz (*Sustiva*) reduces levels of methadone, particularly in the early stages of treatment.

There is conflicting evidence about the effect of using opiates on HIV disease progression, with some studies finding that heroin users progressed to AIDS and death faster, while others did not. Since the advent of anti-HIV treatments, some evidence has emerged that opiate users become resistant to their anti-HIV drugs faster, probably due to poor adherence.

Poppers

Poppers are a nitrite-based drug. Amyl nitrite is used medically to ease the chest pain caused by angina. The drug gets its name from the small glass capsules containing amyl nitrite for the treatment of angina which used to be 'popped' under the nose and inhaled. Amyl and butyl nitrite started to be used recreationally, and have been popular with gay men for many years. More recently, they have become popular with clubbers of all sexualities.

In the UK, poppers are sold in small bottles, which contain a liquid form of butyl nitrite. It is very rare for amyl nitrite to be used as poppers, as its sale is illegal without prescription under the Medicines Act. The legal status of butyl nitrite has been the subject of court cases in recent years. The sale of butyl nitrite poppers is legal, largely because they are sold as 'aromas' or 'room odourisers' rather than as a drug to be inhaled. The possession of poppers, in either amyl or butyl nitrite form, is legal.

When inhaled, poppers cause blood vessels to dilate, allowing more blood to reach the heart. They also cause blood to rush to the brain, speed up heartbeat and relax muscles, providing an intense high lasting a few minutes at most. The drug is widely used to intensify pleasure whilst dancing and having sex. Sniffing poppers relaxes the anal sphincter muscles, allowing anal sex to take place more easily. As poppers dilate blood vessels, many men find that they lose their erection when sniffing them.

After-effects of sniffing poppers may include headache, skin rashes, weakness, sinus pains and burns if the liquid comes into contact with the skin. Sniffing poppers can also cause nausea and vomiting. People with heart or lung problems are advised to avoid poppers, as they can cause breathing problems. In very rare cases, excessive sniffing of poppers can cause the lips and skin to take on a blue tinge. This can be accompanied by vomiting, and shock, and unconsciousness may follow. In extreme cases, deaths have been reported.

The long-term effects of poppers have been a matter of considerable controversy, particularly as it has been argued that their use caused AIDS and particularly Kaposi's sarcoma. However, this view is not supported by any scientific evidence and studies comparing the effects of poppers on HIV-negative and HIV-positive gay men found that only those with HIV suffered any immune damage or progressed to AIDS. However, some animal studies have shown that poppers can suppress immune responses and can have cancer-causing effects. These studies have been criticised because of the relatively large amounts of nitrites given to animals. Any long-term immune damage or cancer-causing effect in humans remains to be proven.

There are no documented interactions between drugs used to treat HIV and poppers. However, sniffing poppers after taking the anti-impotence drugs *Viagra* and *Cialis* can result in a potentially dangerous, even fatal, drop in blood pressure. The dangers from sniffing poppers after taking *Viagra* or *Cialis* are increased if you are also taking a protease inhibitor as part of your HIV treatments. Protease inhibitors cause the amount of *Viagra* or Cialis in the blood to increase, and for this reason it is recommended that people prescribed protease inhibitors take only half the normal dose of *Viagra* or *Cialis* and do not use poppers at the same time.

As with any drug, it may be wise to consider how using poppers affects your wider health and lifestyle, particularly if you are using poppers with other drugs or alcohol. Some people report that using poppers may act as a trigger for unprotected sex and, if this is the case for you, you may wish to have a strategy in place to help you manage this.

Sexual dysfunction drugs

Viagra (sidenafil citrate), *Cialis* (tadalafil) and Levitra (vardenafil) are treatments for erectile dysfunction which have become increasingly popular as recreational drugs, particularly amongst gay men, many of whom use the drug to counteract the impotence side-effect of other recreational drugs such as ecstasy. Several studies have linked use of *Viagra* and *Cialis* with increases in the amount of unprotected sex gay men are having and increased rates of sexually transmitted infections. However, it is unclear if this is because the use of these drugs enables men to have more sexual partners or just increases the amount of sex they are having. It's also possible that men just add the use of anti-impotence drugs to their existing risk-taking repertoire.

The most common side-effect of these anti-impotence drugs is headache. *Viagra, Cialis* and *Levitra* should not be used in conjunction with poppers, as this could cause a potentially dangerous drop in blood pressure.

Protease inhibitors and NNRTIs are metabolised by the body using the same method as *Viagra, Cialis* and *Levitra*, and this can mean that you get very high levels of anti-impotence drugs in your blood, increasing the chances and severity of side-effects. For this reason, you are recommended to reduce by half the standard dose of *Viagra, Cialis* and *Levitra* if you are taking either protease inhibitors or NNRTIs, and not to take more than a single standard dose of either of these impotence drugs in a 48-hour period.

Smoking

Tobacco is a legal and widely used drug. However, smoking is addictive and it is beyond any doubt that smoking can severely damage health and cause early death. HIV-positive smokers may be more likely to get certain AIDS-defining illnesses if they have a weak immune system, and be at increased risk of developing the metabolic side-effects caused by some anti-HIV drugs.

Smoking, in itself, does not make HIV infection worse. The rate at which HIV disease progresses, or at which CD4 cells are lost, is no greater in smokers than non-smokers. Anti-HIV medication is just as effective in smokers as non-smokers.

However, there is very good evidence that people with HIV who smoke are more likely to get certain infections and AIDS-defining illnesses, particularly those affecting the chest. It's known that smokers are approximately three times more likely than non-smokers to develop the AIDS-defining pneumonia PCP. Oral thrush, a common complaint in people with HIV, is also more common amongst smokers.

Emphysema, a smoking-related illness, occurs much more commonly in HIV-positive smokers than HIV-negative smokers.

It's well known that smoking increases the risk of heart disease, high blood pressure, and stroke. It's thought that having a long-term illness like HIV might increase the risk of heart disease. Further, some anti-HIV drugs can cause increases in blood fats, and this can contribute to cardiovascular illnesses. If you smoke and take anti-HIV drugs, then your risks might be increased even further.

It's well established that smoking increases the risk of lung cancer. Although relatively rare, lung cancer seems to occur more often in people with HIV, even if they are taking anti-HIV drugs and have a well-controlled viral load. In one study, all the HIV-positive people who developed lung cancer were smokers.

Stopping smoking (or not starting in the first place) will significantly reduce your risk of developing heart disease and other cardiovascular illnesses. You are most likely to stop smoking and stay stopped if you are motivated.

Individual or group therapy has been shown to help people to stop smoking, and your HIV treatment centre may have a therapy group for individuals who are stopping smoking.

Cigarettes are addictive because they contain nicotine. Many people find that nicotine replacement therapy can help reduce the craving for cigarettes and make quitting easier. Your doctor may be able to prescribe patches, gum, or lozenges which contain nicotine, and there is no evidence that these interact with anti-HIV drugs. You can buy all of them over the counter.

The antidepressant drug bupropion (*Zyban*) has been licensed to help people stop smoking. However, it interacts with anti-HIV drugs of both the protease inhibitor and NNRTI classes, leading to an increase in the amount of bupropion in the blood. Make sure you tell your HIV doctor if you are thinking about taking bupropion. The drug also causes side-effects, including dry mouth, insomnia, headaches, and fits.

Many people find that alternative therapies, such as acupuncture and hypnotherapy, help them stop smoking. Exercise can also be helpful.

Quit is a UK charity which provides help to people who want to stop smoking. Their telephone advice and support service - Quitline - can be reached on 0800 002200. Their website is www.quit.org.uk.

Safer drug use

The importance of safer injecting

HIV can be transmitted by sharing injecting equipment, including water, spoons, needles and syringes. Safer injecting will reduce the chances of you passing on HIV, reduce the chances of you picking up other blood-borne infections, protect you from dirty hits, and protect you from pain and injury when you inject.

Essentials of safer injecting

Get hold of new needles. Find out where there is a needle exchange that provides them free of charge. They will usually offer other services as well.

Always use new needles when you inject. Have a plan to make sure that you have new needles with you when you need them so you never end up sharing needles with others.

Learn how to clean needles. This can be important for situations when you cannot get new needles.

Where to get new needles

Getting free access to new needles differs according to where you live in the UK. Some areas have needle exchanges, others have mobile services, and others have a pharmacy-based service.

Needle exchanges

These are specialist projects set up primarily to exchange used needles and syringes for new ones. They usually offer more than simple needle exchange - sometimes this includes primary health care. Workers in needle exchanges are normally very friendly and non-judgmental.

Mobile or outreach schemes

These are not usually run from a fixed location. These schemes might move from one venue to another, or be housed in a van or bus that visits certain locations at set times, or even be a home delivery scheme.

Pharmacy-based schemes

In some areas, needle exchanges are operated through chemists. Some schemes require minimal registration details, although other are more informal. Even if there is no formal scheme, chemists may sell needles.

How to find needle exchanges

Your HIV clinic will be able to help you. Most needle exchange services will offer safer injecting advice, primary healthcare, safer sex advice, condoms and referrals to other specialist services.

Cleaning injecting equipment

It's best to have a new syringe and needle for every injection. If this is not possible, cleaning your injecting equipment will offer some protection against the transmission of HIV and other infections.

Bleach method

Fill a container with clean, cold water. Draw the water up the needle and fill the syringe, flush out the syringe away from the clean water and repeat. Then fill the container with household bleach, and repeat the cleaning process. Finally, repeat the process again with clean water.

This will kill HIV, provided the bleach is of sufficient strength. Thick bleach can be difficult to draw up a needle, and can also be difficult to flush out, so use thin bleach whenever possible.

Washing-up liquid method

Fill a container with clean, cold water. Draw the water up the needle and fill the syringe, flush out the syringe away from the clean water and repeat. Add a generous squirt of washing-up liquid into another container and dilute with cold water. Repeat the cleaning process, making sure you do not squirt the dirty water into the container with the washing-up liquid. Finally, clean with clean water, using the same process as described above.

Washing-up liquid can kill HIV, but again, thick washing-up liquid can be difficult to draw up fine needles, and bubbles can be left in injecting equipment by this process, so it needs to be thoroughly flushed out before the equipment is used for injecting.

Boiling method

Boiling equipment for five minutes will kill HIV and other infections. However, most disposable syringes will melt if boiled.

Disposing of used injecting equipment

Your local drugs team will be able to tell you about the disposal facilities in your area. Never over-fill containers given to you to dispose of your injecting equipment - two-thirds full is the maximum. With larger syringes, you can put the needle into the barrel of the syringe and push the plunger in until it bends the needle. Put the used equipment in a bag and place in a bin. You can put smaller syringes and needles in a drinks can, crush the can, then put it in a bag and place in a bin.

Dealing with overdose

Reducing the risks of an overdose

The risks of overdosing can be reduced by:

- Being sure of the drug you are injecting.

- Being sure of the strength of the drug supply.

- Not returning to the same dose of a drug after a break, as your tolerance of this drug will have been reduced.

- Not injecting alone or in a place where you cannot be easily found.

- Taking a reduced dose of any new supply.

If you find someone who has taken an overdose:

- Lie the person on their side with their airway clear - this will make sure that they don't choke on their own vomit or suffocate.

- Call an ambulance immediately.

Further reading

- NAM factsheets, *Cannabis, Coccaine, Diarrhoea, Ecstasy, GHB, Immunisations, Ketamine, Methamphetamine, Poppers, Preventing infections,* and *Sleep.*

- *HIV and hepatitis, HIV and sex* and *Nutrition,* booklets in the information for HIV-positive people series produced by NAM.

- 'A healthy lifestyle' in NAM's *HIV and AIDS Treatments Directory.*

- *Protecting you - a basic guide to your immune system,* booklet produced by the Terrence Higgins Trust.

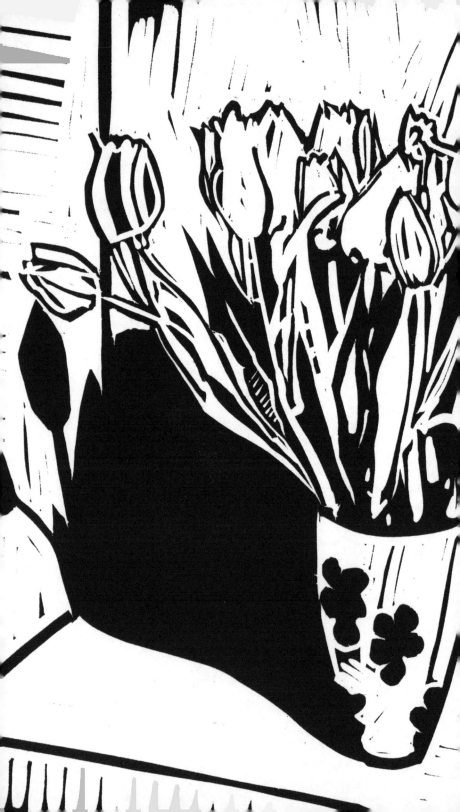

Coping with illness, going into hospital, end of life issues

In this chapter you'll find information on

Some ways to cope with illness.

Some tips on how to manage if you have to go into hospital.

Issues you need to think about if you are terminally ill.

There are testimonies from two men, one writes about his experience of going into hospital for surgery, the other writes about his partner's illness and death and how he responded to it.

Coping with illness

Despite anti-HIV treatments, people with HIV in this country still experience illness. There are about 500 new AIDS diagnoses every year in the UK, and 400 AIDS deaths. This chapter looks at some of the practical things that can be done to make your life easier if you are experiencing illness because of HIV.

In many cases, it will be possible to successfully treat your illness and you'll return to full health. Or it may be that you experience a side-effect, caused by a medicine you are taking, which either goes away or lessens in its severity with time.

However, if you have a very weak immune system and you lose strength, illnesses can become more persistent and harder to fight off, meaning that you need long-term help coping with the effects of illness.

Living an independent life at home can become harder in these circumstances, but there are ways in which you can be assisted to do this. Your local council will have a social services department which will be able to offer a wide range of social care in your own home. Local voluntary organisations can also be helpful offering advice and practical and emotional support. What's available will depend on where you live, and it's important to remember that many local HIV organisations have closed or merged in recent years or have redirected their services towards other areas.

Often, however, it's partners, family, friends or other informal carers who provide the most important support. Informal carers can be put under a lot of practical and emotional strain. They have their own responsibilities to consider, as well as caring for you, and caring for somebody who is ill will inevitably have an emotional impact on them.

The following are key professionals who may provide important services that will allow you to maintain your independence at home during periods of illness.

GPs and primary care

GPs are the only doctors who can visit you in your home. They can also arrange for other health professionals to come to your home, including community nurses. Some hospitals have specialist teams that act as a link between the hospital where you receive your care and local community health services. They can put you into contact with GP and community health services, and sometimes provide direct care themselves.

Community nurses

Community nurses can provide support, help and advice with all the practical aspects of coping with illness and taking medication at home, including changing dressings, looking after an intravenous drip, and taking/giving injections.

They can teach you, or the people looking after you, how to take or give medicines by drip or injection and how to manage some of the problems of illness, such as lifting and bathing. Some community nurses also have specialist skills, for example pain control.

Occupational therapists

Occupational therapists (who are based both in hospitals and in council social services) offer practical ways of improving your quality of life, based on an understanding of your physical and emotional needs and your home environment.

After an assessment involving a detailed discussion of your needs and problems, an occupational therapist will try and work out with you how to solve practical problems at home, how to make tasks easier for you, and how to adapt your home to make it easier to live in and get around.

Palliative care

Palliative care aims to control symptoms and pain and improve quality of life. Palliative care aims to reduce the discomfort and pain of illness (or, indeed treatment side-effects) to a minimum. Some HIV clinics have doctors who are specialists in palliative care or pain control, and there are also nurses, physiotherapists, occupational therapists, dietitians and other members of your healthcare team who can also help.

Going into hospital

There may be times when you need to be admitted to hospital, either to receive a course of treatment for an infection, for surgery, or even to participate in a clinical trial. For most people, going into hospital will be an unsettling, even frightening experience.

When you are first admitted, a nurse will fill out an admission form with you. This will record your name, address, date of birth, next of kin, and religion. You'll also be asked to provide a medical history and say how able you are to look after yourself. If you are having an operation, you'll be asked to give your consent. What an operation involves and why it's being undertaken should be fully explained to you before you give your consent. If anything is unclear, make sure you ask for more information.

Hospital routines can seem very strange. You might find that you have to get up and eat your meals earlier than you are used to doing. You may also feel like you have very little privacy or time to yourself. Ward rounds, medication rounds, consultations with doctors and tests can all feel overwhelming. On top of all this, you'll be away from loved ones and may also have to cope with bad news, illness, pain, or worries over an operation.

You may well see a number of different doctors whilst you're in hospital, and there's a chance that your regular HIV doctor won't be one of them. This can make it harder to ask questions about your treatment and care. If you don't feel able to ask one of your doctors a question, try getting a nurse or other member of the healthcare team to act as an intermediary. Ward rounds, when a group of doctors go from patient to patient can be particularly intimidating. It can be distressing to hear your illness or health discussed as if you weren't there, or as if you were just an interesting problem. Don't be frightened to ask questions during a ward round or remind the doctors that you're there!

Large hospitals are also teaching centres and you may be asked if you can be examined by a medical student as part of their training. It's perfectly okay for you to say no if you are not happy to agree.

If you're admitted to hospital for a reason other than HIV, it would be a good idea to make sure that a doctor or nurse involved in your HIV care knows and liaises with the team providing your care whilst you are in hospital. This will ensure that you receive the right treatment and care.

Visitors
Visitors can really help you cope with a stay in hospital and, particularly on specialist HIV wards, you may find that you're allowed visitors at any time and not just during set visiting hours. But visits can be tiring, particularly if you are feeling unwell, or are weak after an operation or other medical procedure. If you don't feel up to visits, let your friends and family know. The nursing staff on the ward will support any decisions you make about visits.

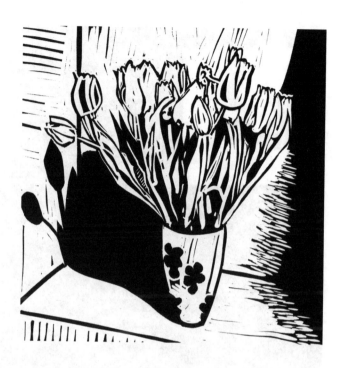

UK Civil Partnerships give registered gay partners the legal right to visit their partner in hospital. Even if you haven't entered into a Civil Partnership you'll almost certainly find that hospitals treat same-sex partners with respect.

Making hospital more comfortable

Having some of your own possessions with you can make a stay in hospital a lot more comfortable and bearable. Some of the most important things you might want to have with you are toiletries, tooth brush and paste, a razor and shaving foam, some clothes to wear during the day, and something to entertain you such as books, magazines and a personal music player. Mobile phones can help keep you in touch, but there may be restrictions on their use on the ward. Having some cash will also probably be useful. Be careful with items of value or money as thefts from patients do occur in hospitals.

Hospital food is often the subject of jokes, and although real efforts have been made to improve it in recent years, you may find it unpalatable. It's okay for visitors to bring food in for you, or for you to order food to be

He was my lover and my best friend. I didn't know how to support him when he tested HIV-positive, and couldn't believe how marvellous his support was when I was diagnosed. I would never have wanted to leave him on his own, but sometimes I wish I had died first, I really miss him now more than ever.

positive voice

delivered to you on the ward. If you're feeling well enough, you may even want to go out for a meal.

Confidentiality

Confidentiality can be an issue during your stay in hospital. It can be hard to conceal that you are HIV-positive if you are staying on a specialist HIV ward and you may want to restrict your visitors to people who already know that you have HIV. Hospital staff shouldn't reveal details about your diagnosis or care to anyone without your consent.

Discharge

You'll be discharged from hospital as soon as you're medically fit. In some circumstances, you may also be discharged into the care of another healthcare provider, such as a hospice.

Before you are discharged, the hospital should do the following:

- Make a follow-up appointment with the appropriate out-patient department. If you were admitted to hospital because of HIV-related causes, this will be at your HIV clinic.
- Give you a telephone number to contact in case of emergencies.
- Give you enough medication to last until your out-patient appointment.
- Ensure that you are able to cope with your medication at home, or that you have help to do so.
- Give you a letter, or discharge note, to give to your GP.
- Arrange for transport to get you home.

End of life issues

Although the prognosis for people with HIV has improved dramatically since the advent of effective anti-HIV treatment, people still die because of HIV. There are some practical issues that you will need to consider if you are facing death soon. These include wills, sorting out your financial affairs, and even funeral choices.

Making a will

Even if you're in perfectly good health, it makes good sense to have a will. A will is the only way of making sure that your partner, family and friends inherit your property in the way you want. Make sure you get a solicitor's advice when drawing up your will. This will ensure that your will is valid. Although it's not advised, you can write your will on forms bought from stationers. Just make sure you appoint an executor (someone to look after your affairs), and that it's signed and witnessed in the presence of two people who won't benefit from the will.

In the UK it is now possible for same sex couples to form Civil Partnerships. These provide the same privileges and responsibilities as heterosexual marriage, including inheritance and next-of-kin rights.

A 'living will'

This is a statement of what kind of medical help you would like to receive if you become seriously ill. It's also called an advanced care directive. It basically sets out what efforts you want doctors to make to try and keep you alive. It also makes clear who you want to make treatment decisions for you if you are unable to do so. A living will can be of great help to the people caring for you, should you ever get this sick.

Power of attorney

If you give someone 'power of attorney', they will be able to sign papers on your behalf when you are unable to do so. You need to see a solicitor to arrange this.

Property

The surviving spouse from a marriage or civil partnership will inherit a property you own should you die. If you are not married to your partner or in a Civil Partnership you should specify that you want your partner to get your property in your will or change the ownership of your property to joint ownership. If you are renting a property with someone, you need to ensure that their name is on the lease along with yours.

Finances

When somebody dies, all their assets are frozen. This includes money in joint bank accounts. This can take some time to sort out after a death, so it's best to plan ahead and make sure that your partner is not dependent on a joint account for access to cash.

If you have a pension or life assurance policy, make sure that you've nominated the person you want to receive benefits from it after your death. If you haven't done this, the company will give the money to your next-of-kin (whatever your will says).

If you have debts, remember that these will pass to your next-of-kin or main beneficiary in your will. If your debts are large, there are some circumstances when bankruptcy might be an option, particularly if you don't own your own home or have a lot of valuable possessions. Places like the Citizens Advice Bureau can tell you what's involved.

Funeral arrangements

If you want, you can arrange this before your death, or you can leave the arrangements to the executor you named in your will. If you haven't made a will, this will pass to your next-of-kin. If you are gay, formally registering your relationship as a Civil Partnership provides an opportunity for your partner to be legally recognised as your next-of-kin. You can say in your will what kind of funeral service you would like, and whether you'd like to be buried or cremated. Funerals can be very distressing occasions for partners, family and friends, and knowing what your wishes were can help make the event less stressful.

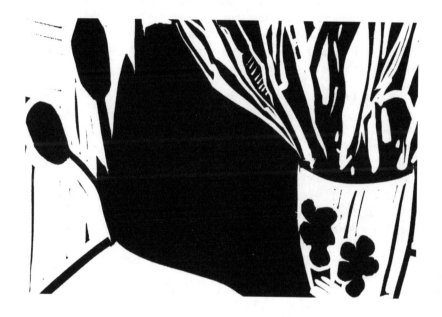

Further reading

- NAM factsheets, *Prognosis*.
- 'Symptoms and illnesses' in NAM's *HIV and AIDS Treatments Directory*.
- *Live long and prosper*, booklet produced by the UK Coalition of People Living with HIV and AIDS.

Billy

1980

When I first met Billy, I was working behind the bar at the Euston Tavern in Kings Cross. Billy had been staring across the bar at me for two months and I hadn't even noticed. Eventually his friends persuaded me to go to a party with them and we ended up standing together in the hall, talking for two hours. I finally realised what was going on - how naïve I was then, a 17-year-old law-breaker (in 1980 the age of consent for gay men was still 21).

1983

We got our first flat together with a borrowed settee, no bed and a fridge that arrived two weeks late.

Home furnishings were never important to Bill; we liked to travel: Barbados, Gambia, America. We saw the world.

1988

A black mark appeared on my leg, starting out as a bruise but turning completely black. It cleared, but if ever my leg scraped against anything these bruises kept appearing.

I visited my GP, who referred me to the local hospital. The consultant I saw suggested that I have a bone marrow test to check my platelet count. It was three.

Panic set in. The consultant seemed quite amazed that I was still breathing. She decided it was time for me to have the big test.

I gave the blood sample and was asked to return in a week. One week later, I was back in the waiting room where I sat. And sat.

Eventually my consultant arrived, looking extremely worried. She confirmed that I had thrombocytopenia, which I already knew. I wanted to know the result of my HIV test.

It took her all her courage to tell me that she had lost the test result and that I would have to give more blood and wait another week. One week later, I had some more news: the blood had been sent somewhere else for "confirmation" and I would have to wait another week for the result.

Week three came and we had a result. To be honest, I really didn't care by then, having been messed around so much. I was positive.

I remember going home; Billy was in the bath and I sat on the toilet next to him and started crying. His only reply was, "thought so - don't worry." Not long after that Billy also tested HIV-positive.

1994

This was our big year: Skiing in France, shopping in New York, partying in Ibiza, lots of weekends away.

Billy was feeling tired in July but still managed to visit the pub every night. He worked in the mornings and slept the afternoons away at home, unless it was sunny, when he would go sunbathing or take the dog to the park.

Trouble started in September, when Billy was made redundant. At the same time he started coughing, a cough that was to be persistent.

Our last holiday together was in Florida in November. Even though Billy was tired, we had a great time together: Disney, MGM, Universal. But on the flight back, Billy said he felt unwell and ended up spending most of the flight in the toilet, trying to cool down.

The first big bomb dropped about three days before Christmas. When we went to the pub together, standing face to face, he said to me, "I know I won't be here this time next year." It was the first negative thing he had said concerning his illness. I remember holding his head, putting it next to mine, and for a brief moment I knew he was telling the truth.

1995

Billy was off on holiday again in the Canaries, this time with a friend from work. I met them at the airport. As soon as I saw them walk through the arrivals door I started crying: Billy looked a shadow of himself (though still the beauty I knew).

In hospital the next day we were told that Billy had a collapsed lung and would have to stay in for a few days. He was determined to get out and go back to Ireland for another break, and told the staff he was going, collapsed lung or not.

Ireland wasn't to be: a filter was put on his lung but on the second day his other lung collapsed. In the course of the next month, both his lungs were operated on. Shortly after his second operation I got a call from a nurse, at 10pm. She said, "Billy can't come to the phone, but can you come up to the hospital now with two tubs of Haagen Daz ice cream?" He picked his moments.

Billy was in hospital for a long time, six weeks of which he was unable to move because of his filters, and we both felt the strain. I was tired, pissed off. I visited some mornings - went to work - back at lunch break - back to work - home to take the dog for a walk before going back to hospital and staying till late. Some nights we didn't even talk.

Although Billy was very frail and exhausted and his weight was down to seven stone, they allowed him home on 11th May.

Within five days, the home care team insisted he should go back to hospital. I dressed him and walked him to the car. He was so thin that on the way to the car his trousers just came down. I was not ashamed.

On the way to the hospital I told him how much I loved him. This was something we always did, but this time I wanted to be sure he knew how much I meant it. He told me it had been a pleasure sharing his life with me. I drove to the hospital in tears.

At the hospital the doctors and nurses were ready for him and a private room had been prepared. Bells started ringing in my head and my body just crumbled; reality was setting in.

I rang a friend and my sister, Kay who, along with the rest of my family, had only known about Billy's illness for two weeks prior to this. Kay arrived and we held each other and cried.

Kay and I stayed on the bed next to Billy, though we didn't sleep. Billy woke twice, once to say he wanted to go home, and once to say he loved me. The morning took so long to arrive.

In the morning my mum arrived. It was so good to see her. Mum, Kay and myself just looked at each other and wept. Billy's sister and brother-in-law arrived in the afternoon, but they didn't want to know what was going on. His sister held Billy but his brother-in-law didn't know what to do.

I hadn't slept for ages, but at around 11.30pm I closed my eyes. I was woken at 12.35am to be told that Billy was going.

How can I ever explain in words how it feels to see someone you love slipping away? Anger, loneliness, emptiness. For the first time in our lives together there was nothing I could do. I remember smelling his hair, his breath, his being. But he was gone.

The care and love of the nurses on the ward was wonderful for Billy and for me and my friends. My friends were incredible and together they saw me through the lowest point of my life.

Until we meet again, Billy, I love you eternally.

Reprinted from the 1996 edition of Living with HIV and AIDS.

Going into hospital
by Christopher

My experiences of hospitalisation are mixed. I've been admitted twice in the last six months, both times for a minor operation. However, following the excellent standards of care I've received at my HIV clinic, I was surprised by my treatment as an in-patient on a general surgery ward.

Before my first operation, my care was exemplary. I attended a pre-surgical outpatient appointment, when I met the surgeon and was examined in preparation for the anaesthetic. On the day of the procedure, a steady stream of nurses, surgeons and anaesthetists visited me on the ward to take information, explain what was going to happen and give me the opportunity to ask any questions.

However, these standards were not maintained once I was back on the ward. It was clear that the nurses were too stretched to offer any care beyond rushing by the bed with the next paper cup of tablets. And as the day wore on, it became obvious that the surgeon was not planning to visit his patients to explain how their procedures had gone, or what to expect over the next few weeks - in my case, the worst pain I have ever experienced.

I was left feeling deeply frustrated. On top of that, I was only told at the last moment that I would have to remain on the ward for three days, rather than being able to go home that evening as promised.

Despite the lack of information, which I do not blame on the staff themselves but on the organisation of the hospital, I was pleasantly surprised by their attitude towards my HIV status (and low CD4 count) and daily visits from my gay partner - although the same could not be said for the other men in the ward, most of whom were over twice my age. I also found the hospital routine less dull than I had imagined - the meals were reasonable, if a little early, and I managed to catch up with some reading and complete a couple of newspaper crosswords. I even popped out for a few pints one evening, with the encouragement of the nurses.

But I came away with a deep resentment of the apparent lack of interest in my needs or wishes after my procedure. Although it is not in my nature, I made an active decision to make a fuss on my second admission, demanding the answers to questions about my treatment and care and questioning the doctors' decisions. This made the experience far more successful and satisfying. Nevertheless, I still left without the promised post-surgical visit from the surgeon, and even without the correct supply of drugs. I eventually saw the surgeon two months later, and was finally given some information about my procedure.

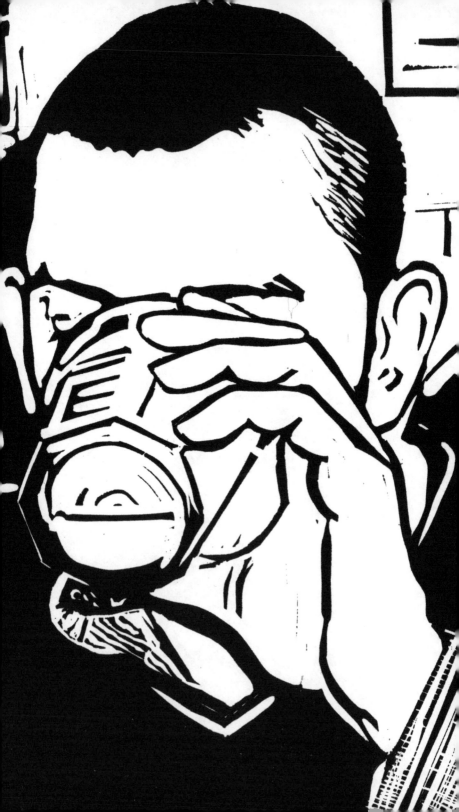

Nutrition and HIV

In this chapter you'll find information on

The importance of a good diet if you
have HIV.

How anti-HIV drugs can affect the types of
food and drink you consume.

Changes to your diet that you may wish to
consider if you experience lipodystrophy,
weight loss, or diarrhoea.

A good diet

Having HIV is unlikely to mean that that you have to make any drastic changes to your diet - your existing diet will probably meet all your nutritional needs. A good diet will consist of a balance of the following items:

Starchy food such as bread, cassava, cereals, banana, millet, maizemeal, potatoes, pasta, rice, and yam. Starchy foods should form the basis of your diet, and will provide carbohydrates for energy as well as vitamins, minerals and fibre. You should eat starchy food at every meal, and have four to six portions each day. A portion is equal to one slice of bread, one medium potato, a bowl of cereal or a cup of rice or pasta.

Fruit and vegetables provide vitamins, minerals, fibre and energy. You should eat five portions a day. A portion is equal to a whole piece of fruit, a heaped serving spoon of vegetables, a small glass of fruit juice, or a handful of dried fruit.

Meat, poultry, fish, eggs, beans nuts provide protein, minerals, and vitamins. Try and eat two or three portions per day. A portion is equal to two medium-sized eggs, a 100g piece of meat, a 150g piece of fish, or a small can of baked beans.

Dairy products such as milk, cheese, and yoghurt provide vitamins, minerals and calcium. Three portions should be eaten per day. A portion is equal to a third of a pint of milk, a small pot of yoghurt, or a matchbox-sized piece of cheese.

Fats such cooking oils, butter, margarine, meat and other protein-based foods provide energy, essential fatty acids and the fat-soluble vitamins A, D, E and K. They also provide calcium and phosphate. It is recommended that about a third of your daily calorie intake should come from fats. But be careful. Eating too much fat can lead to weight gain and increased levels of blood fats. This can increase your chance of developing cardiovascular disease and some cancers.

Dietitians

You can obtain advice on your nutritional requirements from a dietitian. Most HIV clinics have specialist dietitians who can:

- Tell you if your existing diet is meeting all your nutritional requirements.
- Give you advice about any changes in your diet that you may need to make.

- Check your body weight and make sure that your proportion of fat to muscle is appropriate.
- Advise you on any dietary changes you may need to make if you are ill.
- Give you advice on food safety.

Dietitians can also assess your body mass index, a guide to whether your height and weight are in proportion.

Supplements

Many people with HIV take dietary supplements, vitamins, or herbal remedies in the hope of boosting or protecting their immune systems and general health.

Evidence that these have any beneficial effect is somewhat thin. What's more, certain supplements, such as large doses of garlic, can stop some anti-HIV drugs working properly. Most HIV specialists would advise that a healthy, balanced diet is enough to meet your nutritional needs. Megadoses of nutritional supplements are not recommended.

Large doses of vitamin A can cause liver and bone damage, as well as vomiting and headache.

Vitamin C doses above 1,000mg per day can cause kidney stones, diarrhoea and the hardening of the arteries, and have been shown to reduce concentrations of the protease inhibitor indinavir (*Crixivan*).

Zinc doses above 75mg per day have been associated with copper deficiency as well as a shortage of white and/or red blood cells.

Selenium doses of 750 micrograms or more per day have been associated with immune suppression.

Vitamin B6 doses above 2g per day can cause nerve damage, but doses as low as 50mg per day have been known to cause peripheral neuropathy (painful nerve damage), particularly in the feet.

Alcohol in diet

There is no evidence that a couple of alcoholic drinks a day does a person with HIV any harm. Indeed, you might find that a couple of classes of wine or a pint of beer helps reduce stress and anxiety and helps to stimulate your appetite. There's also evidence that a glass or two of alcohol every day can help protect against heart disease.

This isn't an excuse to go out and get roaring drunk every night of the week. Heavy drinking can affect the immune system and slow down recovery from illnesses. Heavy drinking can also cause liver inflammation (hepatitis), and if you have viral hepatitis infections (hepatitis A, hepatitis B, and hepatitis C), you need to talk to your doctor to see if it is safe to drink alcohol at all. The liver plays an important role in processing medicines, particularly drugs used to treat HIV, so it's particularly important to keep your liver healthy if you are HIV-positive.

Alcohol can react badly with some medicines, so whenever you are given a medicine for the first time, ask the pharmacist if it's okay to drink with it.

Food, drink and anti-HIV drugs

Anti-HIV drug combinations may demand one of the following changes to your eating habits:

- Eating at the same time as you take your medication.
- Avoiding food for up to two hours before or an hour after you take your medicines.
- Eating or avoiding certain types of food to ensure that you absorb your medication properly.

When you are prescribed a new medicine, you should be told by your doctor or pharmacist if it has any special dietary restrictions. You should also be given written information explaining what these are.

Detailed information about the dietary restrictions of all the currently available anti-HIV drugs is provided in the NAM booklet *Nutrition*. You can get a free copy from your HIV clinic, or by downloading it from www.aidsmap.com.

Lipodystrophy and diet

Changes in the way the body processes, uses and stores fat have been noticed in some people taking anti-HV drugs. This can lead to changes in body shape or very high levels of blood fats, which can in turn increase the risk of heart disease, stroke and diabetes.

Changes to your diet can help reduce fat levels in your blood (often called lipids). If you are told by your doctor that you have high lipids, try to reduce your intake of saturated fats like dairy products, red meat and animal fats, as well as your sugar and alcohol intake.

Fish oil contains high levels of fatty acids called omega-3 oils, which can reduce fats in the blood. Fish such as mackerel, salmon and trout are a good source. Also, try to make sure that you eat at least five portions of fresh fruit and vegetables a day, as this also protects the heart.

There's a lot more information on lipodystrophy in the chapter *Side-effects*.

Weight loss

When you get ill, you usually lose your appetite. However, when you are ill your nutritional requirements are often increased. Weight loss can be dangerous because it reduces your body's ability to fight off infections and recover.

Dietitians can provide you with some good advice about maintaining your nutritional requirements if you are ill.

Diarrhoea and diet

Diarrhoea is common amongst people with HIV. It can be caused by HIV itself, or by infections or medicines.

Diarrhoea has been reported as a side-effect of all the protease inhibitors, as well as some of the NRTIs and some antibiotics. With some drugs, diarrhoea goes away after the first few weeks of treatment - but some people find that it becomes a permanent feature of living with the drug. The severity of diarrhoea can also differ between people.

Changes of diet seem to have only a limited impact on diarrhoea caused by medicines. But your doctor can prescribe some treatments to help control the diarrhoea. These include:

- Imodium, an anti-diarrhoea drug. It can also be bought over the counter from chemists.

- Calcium supplements have been shown to reduce diarrhoea caused by nelfinavir (*Viracept*).

- Oat bran tablets are also effective against diarrhoea caused by medicines. They work by absorbing fluid and slowing the movement of stool through the gut.

If you have bad diarrhoea, you are likely to lose valuable nutrients. Eating bananas, chicken and fish can help restore levels of potassium which are commonly depleted in people with bad diarrhoea. Avoid coffee, raw vegetables and spicy food as these can make diarrhoea worse.

Further reading

- *Anti-HIV drugs*, and *Nutrition*, booklets in the information for HIV-positive people series produced by NAM.

- 'Anti-HIV therapy' in NAM's *HIV and AIDS Treatments Directory*.

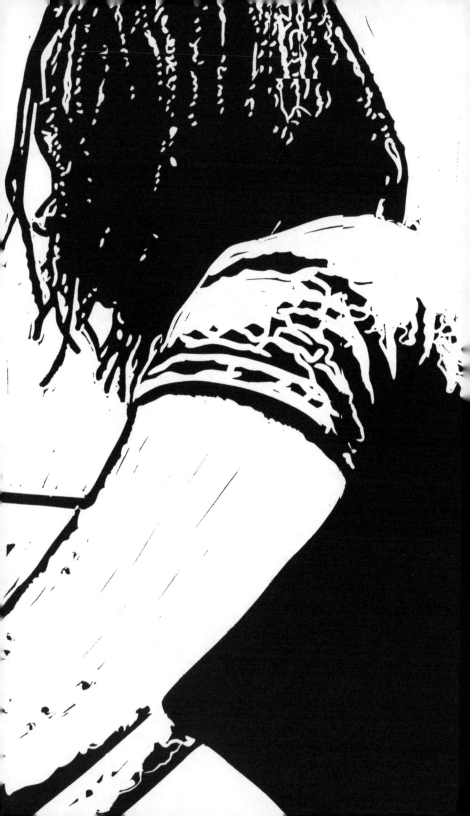

Exercise

In this chapter you'll find information on

The benefits of exercise.

How to plan for and sustain exercise.

Exercise and diet and the use of
anabolic steroids.

A man writes about his participation in
an endurance event following his
HIV diagnosis.

Benefits of exercise

Everyone can benefit from some form of exercise and experience a lift to their overall health and well-being. Moderate exercise is beneficial to the immune system, and can also improve mood and offer an important way of maintaining a healthy self-image.

Aside from popular forms of exercise like swimming, cycling, aerobics, running and weight training (sometimes called resistance training), there are a number of movement-based exercises, such as yoga, which help maintain muscle tone and suppleness whilst also having meditative or relaxing qualities.

Blood lipids are the name given to fatty substances in the blood, such as cholesterol and triglycerides. Having high levels of these substances in the blood raises your risk of coronary heart disease. Taking anti-HIV drugs may lead to raised blood lipids.

Raising the heart rate for at least thirty minutes three times per week through aerobic exercise (such as cycling, running, swimming, or even brisk walking) reduces these fats, and so lowers risk of heart disease.

People with HIV-related wasting often have low levels of a type of cholesterol called HDL; sometimes referred to as 'good' cholesterol. Resistance training has been shown to significantly increase HDL cholesterol in HIV-positive men with normal testosterone levels.

Regular exercise has been shown to reduce total body and trunk fat among HIV-positive men with body fat changes (lipodystrophy). Resistance exercise reduces raised triglycerides and cholesterol levels.

Planning for exercise

Think about what your aims of exercising are and set yourself some realistic and achievable goals. You may want to get fitter, or you may want to put on weight, lose weight, or achieve a better body shape. Make sure that your aims are achievable - if you're too ambitious you might become disappointed and lose enthusiasm for your exercise programme, or, at worst, injure yourself.

Getting an instructor at a gym to work with you to develop a personal training programme can be a good way of setting yourself achievable goals. Many gyms offer this service as part of an induction package for members.

Make sure that you tell the person working with you about any health conditions you have that might make exercise risky (for instance, high blood pressure) or which affect your ability to undertake certain exercises, such as a sprained ankle. There's no reason why you have to tell anybody at a gym or other fitness facility that you are HIV-positive.

Types of exercise

There are two types of exercise. Aerobic exercise (oxygen burning), and resistance (weight training). You're likely to experience the best results with a training programme that incorporates both these types of exercise.

Aerobic exercise

Aerobic exercise improves your heart's ability to pump and your muscles' ability to use oxygen. It includes activities like brisk walking, running, cycling, and swimming.

Aerobic exercise should be strenuous enough to make you out of breath but still able to talk. A total of 30 minutes of aerobic activity per day will reduce your risk of heart disease. If you maintain your heart rate within a training range for 20 to 30 minutes three times a week, you will improve your fitness level. It is easy to calculate your training heart rate. You should aim to exercise between 60% - 75% of your maximum heart rate.

To find your maximum heart rate subtract your age from 220, e.g. 220 - 39 = a maximum heart rate of 181. Multiply 181 by 0.6 to get the lower end of your training heart rate and by 0.75 to get the upper end. Therefore, the training heart rate of a 39 year-old is between 109 and 139 beats per minute.

Resistance training

The most efficient way to improve your muscle strength and size is through resistance or weight training. Activities like swimming and yoga provide some resistance, but the most efficient way is to use free weights or weight machines at a gym. To improve muscle strength, you need to overload the muscle. This involves doing quite a small number of repetitions using relatively heavy weights. You should be able to go three sets of 8-12 repetitions. As your strength improves, increase the weight. Always stretch and warm up before exercise. This helps reduce the risk of injury. Don't overdo things. You risk hurting yourself.

People with bleeding disorders should consult their doctor before embarking on a programme of resistance training. Tearing muscles during resistance training can cause internal bleeding that can leave the muscle permanently damaged. People with haemophilia should take Factor VIII if they are weight training.

Sustaining exercise

It's likely that you'll have a high level of enthusiasm when you start your new exercise programme, but this may well diminish in the weeks and months that follow. Exercising can be boring, tiring and uncomfortable. But there are some easy steps you can take to make it easier on yourself:

- It doesn't have to be a chore. Nobody is forcing you to do this. Remember, you are doing it because you want to.

- Choose an exercise activity that you enjoy. There's no point doing something that you don't like. Similarly, if you are going to a gym, choose one that you feel comfortable using.

- Set goals that are achievable, and record your progress.

- Try to prioritise exercise. Don't treat it as a peripheral activity.

- Try and exercise with other people. Becoming a member of a running, swimming or other sporting club can be a great way of exercising with people. Don't feel intimidated - there will be members of all abilities.

- Don't punish yourself or feel guilty if you miss a session or do less than you hoped. You can always go back another day.

- Don't exercise if you are ill or feel unwell. It will probably do you more harm than good.

- Vary your exercise routine.

- Allow yourself regular days off. Your body needs time to recover and benefit from exercise. If you've been exercising regularly, an annual two-week holiday with no exercise won't do you any harm at all.

Fuel for exercise

Before the workout begins, ensure that you are properly hydrated. During each workout, ensure that you maintain an adequate fluid intake. You should try to drink at least 150ml to 250ml every 15 minutes during a session - but if you are taking the protease inhibitor indinavir (*Crixivan*), increase this slightly, to protect against kidney stones.

You're likely to find it uncomfortable if you exercise before breakfast, or immediately after a large meal. The best time to exercise is 30 minutes after a light snack or a meal replacement drink. Do not eat during a workout, but do try to eat a meal high in carbohydrate and protein as soon as possible after each session, in order to promote muscle tissue growth. Seek advice from a registered dietitian at your treatment centre on developing a suitable diet plan.

Steroids

Anabolic steroids can, in certain circumstances (such as severe muscle wasting), be prescribed by your doctor as a way of improving energy levels and enhancing the effects of exercise.

If you are experiencing weight loss, anabolic steroids might a way of combating this. Talk to your doctor about whether they would be an appropriate treatment for you.

Many people use anabolic steroids which they have bought illegally, to boost the effects of training at the gym. You should be aware that there are many different kinds of steroids, of differing quality, strength and availability, and that inappropriate use can lead to severe liver damage.

Further reading

- NAM factsheets, *Cholesterol, Exercise* and *Lipodystrophy*.
- *Nutrition,* booklet in the information for HIV-positive people series produced by NAM.
- *Are you living well with HIV?* and *Feel good, take control, stay healthy,* leaflets produced by the Terrence Higgins Trust.
- *In gear: a gay man's guide to steroids,* booklet produced by Camden and Islington's Gay Men's Team, 020 7530 3922.

Ironman

My diagnosis for HIV occurred just after I'd entered the first UK Ironman triathlon (an incredibly strenuous event that involves a long swim and cycle ride followed by a full marathon) scheduled to be held in August 2005 and I was just in the process of ramping up my training regime. I was now wondering whether or not I'd be able to complete this dream in view of my HIV diagnosis. But I was inspired by Jane Tomlinson, who is terminally ill with cancer who'd successfully completed the Florida Ironman in 2004.

After taking a couple of weeks off from training in February 2005 to reflect, I decided I was going to go for it and got back into heavy training for the next seven months. I also told my boss at work who was supportive and I knew I could trust. With him aware of my HIV status I felt more comfortable. Should I have problems in the future at least he's be sympathetic. The only people I've told are my best mate and GP.

In August I completed the Ironman in 13 and a half hours - given I had torn my calf muscle two weeks before the event I was pretty pleased with my achievement.

It's now January 2006, and my CD4 count is steady - at just over 350, though they did dip to 251 earlier this month due to a cold. I'm not yet on anti-HIV medication. I'm pretty confident that my healthy lifestyle (okay, I know I smoke the odd cigarette, but I will give up soon, I promise!) and constantly improving anti-HIV drugs will keep me around for quite some time yet.

I'm optimistic about the future and have entered another Ironman which will take place in July 2006.

Mental health

In this chapter you'll find information on

The now rare HIV-related mental disorders.

Mental health problems such as distress,
depression and anxiety.

Mental health side-effects of
anti-HIV drugs.

Four men write about their experiences of
mental health problems.

Mental health problems can affect anybody, but it seems that people with HIV are more likely to experience a range of mental health problems, not least because the groups most affected by HIV in the UK, gay men, refugees and migrants and drug users, are already more likely to have mental health problems. Advanced HIV infection itself is known to cause mental health problems, although these are now very rare. More common are feelings of acute emotional distress which often accompany adverse life-events and clinical mental disorders such as depression and anxiety. In addition, some anti-HIV drugs can cause psychological disturbance.

HIV-related mental disorders

It is estimated that before anti-HIV treatments became widely used, 7% of people with advanced HIV infection would develop dementia. Mania has also been observed in people with advanced HIV disease. It is highly unusual for a person who has been treated with anti-HIV drugs to develop either of these conditions as a direct result of being HIV-positive.

Symptoms of dementia include:

- Difficulty in thinking or understanding, such as forgetfulness, loss of memory, loss of concentration and confusion.
- Changes in behaviour, including loss of interest, feelings of isolation and childishness.
- Problems with movement and coordination, such as loss of balance or strength from the limbs.

There can be many causes of the symptoms listed above, including depression and infections, as well as dementia. So, it's very important to see your doctor to find out what the real cause is.

Some anti-HIV drugs appear to offer protection against the development of dementia. The first anti-HIV drug seen to help prevent dementia developing and as a treatment for the condition was AZT (zidovudine, *Retrovir*). More recently, d4T (stavudine, *Zerit*) and abacavir (*Ziagen*) have also been shown to offer protection against dementia and to help prevent the condition. A study has also suggested that combinations containing efavirenz (*Sustiva*) may be effective.

The reason why only some of the currently available anti-HIV drugs work against dementia is because the brain and spine are separated from the blood by the blood-brain barrier, which only allows very small molecules to get into the central nervous system. AZT, d4T, abacavir and efavirenz's effects on dementia are thought to be due to their ability to cross the blood-brain barrier, achieve effective levels and fight HIV in the brain. Some researchers argue that any anti-HIV regimen that significantly improves the immune system should also improve dementia, as immune cells can cross the blood-brain barrier.

Emotional distress

Particular events such as receiving an HIV diagnosis, bereavement, the break down of a relationship, financial worries or work problems, or dealing with side-effects of treatment can result in feelings of deep unhappiness and emotional distress which are difficult to manage and interfere with a person's ability to get on with daily life.

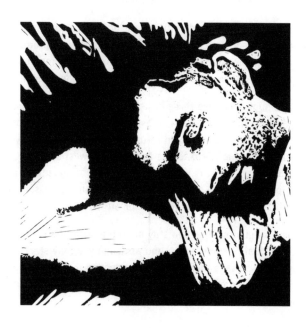

Support from family and friends can be very helpful at these times, as can professional help, such as helplines and counselling. Many HIV clinics have specialist mental health teams and some HIV support agencies can offer short courses of counselling. Some people also find that complementary therapies, such as acupuncture, can relieve some of the symptoms of emotional distress, although these are now rarely provided by HIV clinics.

Depression

Depression is a clinical illness and is twice as common in people with HIV as in the general population.

Depression can be triggered by illness or social problems, but it is not uncommon for there to be no readily identifiable cause. It is characterised by the presence of most or all of the following symptoms on a daily basis for several weeks: low mood; apathy; poor concentration; irritability; insomnia; early waking or oversleeping; inability to relax; weight gain or weight loss; loss of pleasure in usual activities; feelings of low self-worth; excessive guilt; and recurrent thoughts of death or suicide.

If you are diagnosed with depression, your doctor may recommend that you take antidepressant drugs, which relieve the symptoms of depression by altering chemicals in the brain which influence mood and behaviour. They can take several weeks to work and may have side-effects.

Although there are three classes of antidepressant drugs used (tricyclics; MAOIs; and SSRIs), it is most likely that you will be offered a drug from the SSRI (selective serotonin re-uptake inhibitors) class, which includes drugs like fluoxetine (*Prozac*), as these have fewest side-effects and interactions with other drugs. It is not uncommon for drugs in this class to cause sexual problems. You must not take the herbal antidepressant St John's wort if you are taking a protease inhibitor or an NNRTI.

The amount of time you stay on antidepressants will depend on your individual circumstances, and although you may start to feel better soon after starting to take them, it is recommended that you remain on them for at least three months if it is your first depressive illness, or longer if your depression has recurred.

Mental health problems as a side-effect of anti-HIV treatment

It is known that the anti-HIV drug efavirenz can cause psychological disturbances. Some people have difficulty sleeping, or vivid dreams or nightmares. Other people have reported depression without any other apparent cause.

Anxiety

Anxiety is a feeling of panic or apprehension, which is often accompanied by physical symptoms such as sweating, rapid heart beat, agitation, nervousness, headaches and panic attacks. Anxiety can accompany depression or be seen as a disorder by itself, often caused by circumstances which result in fear, uncertainty or insecurity.

If anxiety is caused by practical problems, then getting advice, talking the problem through or counselling might be helpful. Anxiety which accompanies

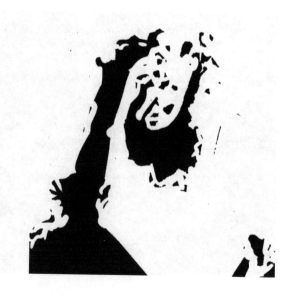

depression is relieved by antidepressant drugs. Some people find massage or other complementary therapies help relieve the symptoms of anxiety.

Drugs such as benzodiazepines, including *Valium*, are now very rarely prescribed as a treatment for long-term anxiety because they are addictive. However, they are still used in the treatment of short periods of acute anxiety without any long-term dependency problems.

Talking therapies

Often drug therapies for mental problems work better if accompanied by talking therapies designed to help people understand and control their feelings. Examples include psychotherapy and cognitive behavioural therapy (CBT), both of which usually involve a short course of sessions with a psychotherapist or psychologist.

Further reading

- NAM factsheets, *Dementia*, *Mental health* and *Sleep*.
- *Adherence*, *Anti-HIV drugs* and *Mental Health*, booklets in the information for HIV-positive people series produced by NAM.
- 'Symptoms and illnesses' in NAM's *HIV and AIDS Treatments Directory*.
- 'Mental health and quality of life' in NAM's *HIV and AIDS Reference Manual*.
- *Depression* leaflet produced by the Terrence Higgins Trust.
- *Getting ready* and *Getting what you want*, booklets produced by PACE and Camden and Islington Gay Men's Team.

A permanent feature

Depression has become a more or less permanent feature of my life with HIV. I used to get depressed before my HIV diagnosis - at times I've wondered if the main reason I ended up contracting HIV was because I'd been spent so much of my adolescence and young adulthood depressed.

It wasn't that I didn't know about HIV - I could have written a small book on the subject - but I just didn't have the emotional nounce and assertiveness to put that knowledge into practice.

My first experience of depression was when I was 17. I was revising for my 'A' levels at the time and I put down the feeling of hopelessness that enveloped me that early spring to worry about exams. Well, I'm sure that concern about getting the grades to get a place at university was making me anxious, but there was something else causing my contributing to my growing sense of despair and hopelessness. I knew I was gay, and, sorry if this isn't PC, I didn't like it.

It wasn't a good time to realise you were gay. AIDS was just starting to become a big news story and was being called the 'gay plague' by the tabloids. The then Conservative government was in the process of passing Section 28, banning local councils from 'promoting' homosexuality, the chief constable of the Greater Manchester Police, in whose jurisdiction I lived, had said that gay men only had themselves to blame for AIDS, his 'direct line' to God telling him that gay men were 'wallowing in filth of their own making.'

For years I'd been called a 'poof' or 'queer' by other kids at school because I was crap at football and looking back on it I know that I was different. I did my best to keep my head down and not to attract too much attention, but it didn't make much difference and I gradually came to dislike myself for being who I was. The school I went to was quite religious and although I can't really remember the teachers there saying anything about gays or homosexuality, it was made very clear that any sex outside marriage was sinful. I can remember praying every night, asking God to stop making me fancy the boy who sat next to me. It didn't work. I then used to ask myself, 'why me?'

My Mum and Dad were very loving, but they used to make constant remarks about actors like Dirk Bogart being 'queer' and I didn't feel I could turn to them for support. Nor could I tell any of my friends - jokes about puffs made that clear.

I got through my bout of depression, sailed through my 'A' levels and secured my place at university in London. I made a small number of friends in my first year, but didn't tell any of them that I was gay. I tried to ignore it myself and worked really hard, and just drank myself into oblivion whenever it became something I thought about - I lost count of the times I got so drunk I couldn't remember what I'd done the night before.

Finally, I realised I had to do something about it and told a female friend I was gay. She encouraged me to go to a gay bar in King's Cross. Well, after walking past it several times I finally plucked up the courage to go in. It was really exciting, full of happy people having fun. Lots of the men were very sexy. But none of them seemed interested in me. I got very drunk.

A sort of pattern emerged. I didn't feel that I belonged in the straight world, nor did I really feel I belonged on the gay scene either. This was mainly because I just didn't feel desirable. I focused on my every fault. Everybody seemed to be having so much fun, except me.

Well, I kept on drinking, and when I wasn't drinking I was in the library. This carried on for a few years. I got a good degree, and a well paid job. But I was desperately unhappy. I don't think I knew what it would take to make me happy. I'd made a few gay friends, but my connection to them seemed very superficial. There was no way I could tell them that I didn't actually like being gay.

My life just seemed rubbish, and I'd regularly slip into black moods. My sleep would become worse, I'd get irritable, feel sorry for myself, say things like 'I hate myself' whilst looking in the mirror - or even whilst walking down the street when I remembered something that distressed me. I can remember asking myself if there was any point to life, and the answer was 'no'. Thoughts of killing myself started to enter my mind. I really remember walking along the Embankment and thinking how easy it would be just to jump in the river.

And then things would brighten. Life wouldn't seem so bad after all. It was in one of these bright moments that I met my first boyfriend, Jed, at the cheese counter at my local super market. We hit it off. He made me feel really good about myself. He gave me HIV. I don't blame him at all. He didn't have a clue he had it. I can remember that I really didn't want to have unsafe sex but just didn't know how to say no, I couldn't stand up for myself.

Actually, my mood didn't immediately get worse when I found out I had HIV. If anything, it lightened. I just sort of gave up caring. I packed in my job and went on benefits. Things were alright for a year or so. But then I started to notice a predictable pattern in my mood occurring. I started to feel bad about the way I looked and for being who I was, telling myself that I'd ruined my life and was a terrible failure. Just look at the evidence - I couldn't even stop myself getting HIV. Jed and I had split up and I was going out a lot. But nobody seemed interested and drink was the only real companion I had on nights out. Gradually I started slipping into cycles of depression. The intervals between the depressions got shorter and the episodes of depression started to last longer and become more intense.

Eventually I asked for some help from my doctor. He put me on *Prozac* and sent me to see a head doctor. I've been on *Prozac* ever since.

I have got on with my life. I've got a job, I'm doing okay on HIV medication. But most of the time I'm really unhappy. Sometimes I have thoughts that really make me ashamed. I'm probably not allowed to say things like this - but I sort of wish that HIV treatment had never come along, I'd probably be dead my now and all my worries would be over. But then, my mood brightens again, and yes, I am glad to be alive and still have years of life left.

Trouble is, I don't have a clue what to do with them. I feel so alone. Who'd want to be with somebody with HIV? I was never an oil painting to start with and that's got worse since I got side-effects from my HIV drugs.

Life is a struggle - I'm trying to sort out why I have such bad feelings about myself - I tell myself that it's because I grew up in such an anti-gay environment and always felt like an outsider. But I don't really believe that - I just feel like a freak a lot of the time and that I don't deserve love or acceptance. At times like that it seems quite fitting that I have HIV.

But the fact that I do struggle does mean something. It means that I'm not prepared to put up with the rubbish. That I really do, deep down, believe that I deserve better. If I start loving myself, then perhaps somebody will love me, HIV and all. I think that's a good place to stop writing.

Alone, by John

I cannot tell my family that I have HIV as I am afraid of losing them.

As for a relationships or love, well that seems impossible. Meeting guys in a small northern town isn't quite as easy as it is living in London or Manchester.

I live in poverty, isolation and loneliness. I have mental health problems, and lack self-esteem and confidence. I really do feel that I no longer have control over my destiny.

Coping, by Frank

I started to write about my experiences of learning to cope with HIV some time ago. The unpleasant memories it forced me to recall upset me so much I had to take a break.

I was diagnosed with HIV in March 1991 after several months of ongoing severe flu-like symptoms. HIV wasn't much spoken of then and I wasn't really aware of it. Nor did I really think that I was at any real risk.

For the past year I'd been in a relationship which had recently ended after months of violence - including forced sex. My partner had not told me that he was HIV-positive and I'd not picked up on any clues to suggest that he might have HIV.

The disappointment and frustration of the relationship break-up had left me emotionally exhausted and physically weak. It was only some months later that I considered the possibility of HIV and asked my doctor for an HIV test, which was positive.

The consultant I was referred to was very supportive, and gave me time to ask questions. I pressed him for an indication of my prognosis, and he said that I could probably expect to live for another two years.

On the basis of this information, I made a will, distributed most of what I owned to family and others - and waited.

Fortunately I had some very good friends who I could confide in, and talking things over with them was the single greatest support I had during those awful months. It was a great relief just to be with them doing simple things, comfortable that they knew and understood me and what I was going through.

Gradually, I got stronger and was able to resume living a life and socialising. I began to enjoy each day as it came. I read a lot, and went away for holidays.

My friends knowing that I had HIV made a great difference. It meant that I could opt out of arrangements, leave dinner parties early, and, when I was on holiday, rest without people being offended. I could also take my medicines without explanation or embarrassment. That's not to say I was a total bore - I did make an effort.

There were still some bad times when medicines caused serious side-effects. I tried to remove stress from my life by lightening my work-load and responsibilities.

There was also a void in my life - a lack of physical and emotional intimacy. For five years I was celibate.

Then, nine years after my diagnosis, I met my partner, Michael, and we have been very happy ever since. It helped that he knew my status from the start. We met with my consultant together and discussed my health. I believe firmly that his support and understanding, his affection and love have been the main factor in my well-being. His very interest in my health and well-being has been life-enhancing for me.

The medical staff, my family, friends and partner have each played their own invaluable, unique and greatly appreciated part in my survival for so long with HIV, and have wonderfully enriched my life.

Russ

It is about nine years since I was told I was HIV-positive and it is almost the same amount of time since I met my partner, Chris, and started a stable relationship. These statements seem to run in tandem but the paths between them have been anything but smooth. My story is about denial, emotional feelings and the role that HIV can play in the creation and development of personal relationships. It is, in short, a truthful account of the emotional difficulties I have encountered which you may have empathy with.

My partner Chris is HIV-negative and has been well throughout the whole period, but I must go back to the start of August 1995 to begin my story.

Being HIV-positive and single seemed natural. This hidden, awful virus did not exactly make me feel good about myself. The doctors were telling me I had only a few years to live, so somehow the idea of searching for a partner seemed futile. If I had only a short time to live, I certainly did not see any benefit in using up time and energy on emotional issues. Instead, I went out drinking nearly every night, and slept around, worked hard, socialised a lot and tried to enjoy every minute of the day. I remember feeling very tired, but put that down to HIV, and not my lifestyle. When illness came, I would enlist the support of members of the caring professions. Single, free, happy and busy, with a back-up. I really thought I had it all worked out. Maybe you have felt that, or perhaps you feel it now, and there is no doubt it is a nice feeling. Then one evening, at the start of one of my drinking binges, I met Chris. I was buzzing and felt confident and happy. One of the first things he said to me was that I had sad eyes. In one second, my whole life seemed to stop in the face of such directness. I felt the need to retaliate, and told him I was HIV-positive very much in the vein of "take that". The response? A kiss of passion and the word "So?"

So Chris entered my life when I did not want anyone. For me, facing up to HIV meant addressing the emotional as well as the medical issues. In short, it was permissible for me to love someone and even more important for someone to love me. Some of you will be laughing or sneering about this, perhaps - but remember at the time I am talking about, 1995, the life expectancy of most people living with HIV was quite short.

Now I was starting to feel emotions and that should have been good, but it did not work that way. I felt sad, hopeless and anxious, and furthermore I felt lonely. How could I be lonely when I was living with my partner? Then I felt envious of his good health and thought about how I had once been. A few years into the relationship, I was a mess and was being treated for depression. You see, this is no Hollywood love story. The recovery does come, or else I would not be writing this, but it was difficult. It involved long-term counselling and a hell of a lot of effort on the part of Chris and myself. In short, I learned to involve myself in Chris's life and found my self-identity again as Russ, not Russ who is HIV-positive.

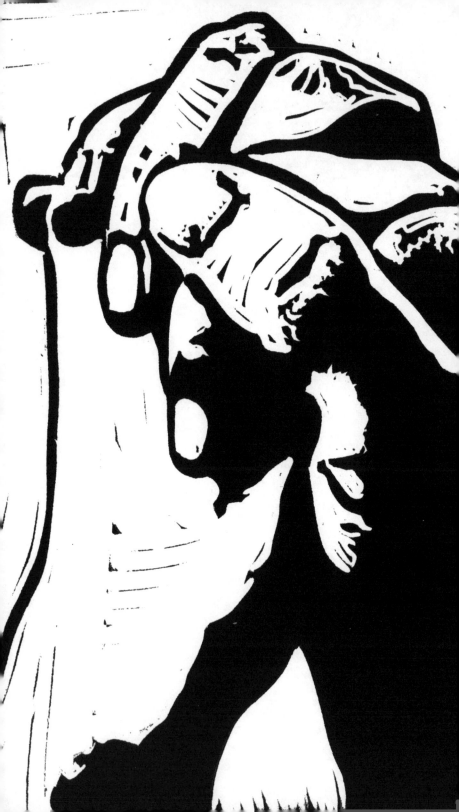

Sex

In this chapter you'll find information on

How finding out you have HIV might affect
your attitudes towards sex.

Some strategies to help you deal with
sexual problems.

The importance of good sexual health and
sexual health check-ups.

How HIV is transmitted and how you
can protect your own and other people's
sexual health.

Why an undetectable viral load doesn't
necessarily mean that you aren't infectious.

Reinfection with other strains of HIV.

One man writes about his experiences of
anal warts; another writes about how his
experiences of sex since his HIV diagnosis
and another writes about a sexual
encounter with a man whose HIV status he
does not know.

HIV sex and you

Although it's not certain to happen, you may find that your feelings about sex change after you find out you have HIV. It could be that your interest in sex dips or goes away altogether for some or all of the time, or the opposite might happen. This could be due to natural fluctuations in your desire for sex and is something that you are prepared to put up with but. Alternatively, it could cause you problems, particularly if it makes you unhappy or interferes with other aspects of your life.

Finding out you have HIV can make you feel differently about yourself. It may well be a shock and may result in you going off sex, at least temporarily. Some people say that having HIV makes them feel less physically and sexually desirable and they lose confidence dating or with their sexual partners.

Having HIV can make you to look at yourself and sex very negatively. It could make you feel bad about the kind of sex you had or are having, make you worry about the risk of infecting somebody else with a potentially fatal illness, or make you angry with the person or people who could have infected you.

An HIV diagnosis might also feed wider negative feelings you have about who you are. HIV has been used as a moral and political tool to criticise and stigmatise the groups most affected in this country - gay men, Africans and drug users.

It is important to remember that HIV is an infection - it is not a moral judgment or a punishment.

Anxiety about infecting sexual partners with HIV is also common and this can mean that your desire to have sex or your sexual performance dips.

An additional source of anxiety may be telling your past, present or potential sexual partners that you have HIV. This can be daunting and you need to decide yourself whether you tell none, some or all of your sexual partners.

Infecting somebody with HIV after having unprotected sex could have serious legal implications. See the chapter, *HIV and the Law*.

Think about how and when you are going to tell people that you have HIV, and how you would react if somebody rejected you. Although many HIV-positive people have HIV-negative long-term partners or casual partners, people are rejected because they have HIV. It can hurt (or even in some circumstances put your personal safety at risk) and it is important that you develop strategies to cope if this happens to you.

Many HIV-positive people have partners who are HIV-negative. Many couples are able to have protected sex all the time, but others find this difficult or impossible and are willing to accept the risk of the uninfected partner contracting HIV. In some circumstances power imbalances in a relationship can mean that even though one partner wants to have safer sex, the other partner insists that condoms are not used.

HIV can also lead to a loss of sexual intimacy in relationships. Enjoying and valuing intimacy in ways other than sex might be valuable if this occurs.

Some HIV-positive people choose only to have sex with people who also have HIV - this is sometimes called 'serosorting'. This can be motivated by a wish not to risk infecting a partner with HIV. Another reason might be a wish to have unprotected sex with other HIV-positive people. This can be pleasurable and intimate, but there can be health risks including sexually transmitted infections, infection with hepatitis C and possible reinfection with another strain of HIV. These issues are discussed in greater detail in the following pages.

Dealing with sexual problems

Whilst sexual dysfunction can be a problem for anyone, people living with HIV may be particularly affected. Loss of sexual drive or desire (libido) can have a significant impact on quality of life and feelings of self-worth, and may contribute to emotional problems such as anxiety and depression.

Sexual problems are common during times of stress, such as when one receives an HIV-positive diagnosis. This can be a time of shock, worry, and disbelief and sexual desire and performance can suffer as a result. Concerns about possibly infecting your sexual partners can also affect sex and intimacy. Negative associations between HIV - a potentially life-threatening infection - and sex could also cause sexual problems.

Other everyday issues can also affect sexual desire and performance, for example work or relationship difficulties. If they do not go away, ask for help.

Excessive intake of alcohol or recreational drugs can also diminish both the desire and ability to have sex.

Many of the drugs commonly used to treat depression, e.g. fluoxetine (*Prozac*) or paroxetine (*Seroxat*) can also affect sexual function.

Additionally, megestrol acetate (*Megace*), an appetite stimulant, has been shown to cause loss of libido.

Sexual dysfunction among men can often be a result of decreased testosterone levels (hypogonadism), which can also lead to fatigue. Lower than normal testosterone levels have been found in people with advanced HIV infection, and can be caused both by the direct effects of HIV or chronic ill health itself. Many men receive testosterone treatment to alleviate these problems. Men who use testosterone replacement therapy usually gain muscle mass, experience an emotional 'lift', and an increase in their libido.

Impotence, or the inability to get or maintain an erection, can be caused by HIV damaging the nerves in the penis that control an erection (this is called autonomic neuropathy). Similarly, anti-HIV drugs that cause neuropathy such as ddI (didanosine, *Videx/Videx EC*) and d4T (stavudine, *Zerit*) may cause numbness in the genital area, which can make it difficult to sustain an erection. Protease inhibitors have also been reported to cause impotence, with some evidence suggesting that those containing ritonavir are particularly likely to cause sexual dysfunction.

Don't be ashamed if you're not happy with the way you feel about sex or about your sexual performance. Try talking to your partner or a close and trusted friend about what you are feeling or experiencing. Your HIV doctor will help or refer you to a specialist, nurse, health advisor or counsellor who can. If it is a medicine which is causing your sexual problems it might be possible to change it to one that does not have these side-effects. It is also possible that your doctor might be able to refer you to a specialist HIV counsellor where you will have an opportunity to talk through your concerns and problems. In other cases a referral to specialist HIV mental health services might be appropriate. Here you may be offered a course of cognitive behavioural therapy (CBT) to help you recognise and over-come your sexual problems.

Medicines may also be able to help. The drugs sildenafil (*Viagra*), tadalafil (*Cialis*) and vardenafil (*Levitra*) are tablets used to treat impotence which works by increasing blood flow to the penis, making it more sensitive to touch. However, these drugs should be taken with care by people using protease inhibitors, non-nucleoside analogues (NNRTIs), the anti-fungal drug ketoconazole (*Nizoral*), itraconazole (*Sporanox*) or the antibiotic erythromycin. For people taking full-dose ritonavir (*Norvir*), it is recommended that *Viagra* should not be used at all given the potential health risks. Similarly, the recreational drug poppers must not be used with *Viagra*, *Cialis*, or *Levitra* under any circumstances as this can result in a dangerous drop in blood pressure.

HIV sex and the law

See the section, 'HIV and the law: HIV transmission and the criminal law'.

Sexual health

Sexual health is important to everybody, but is especially important if you have HIV because sexually transmitted infections (often shortened to STIs) can not only cause illness, but increase the chances of you passing on HIV during unprotected sex, even if you have an undetectable viral load.

Although sexually transmitted infections can seem minor, they can and do cause unpleasant symptoms. If left untreated, some can cause severe health problems. In the very long-term, some can cause irreversible damage and in extreme cases, be fatal.

Some sexually transmitted viral infections, such as herpes simplex virus -2 (HSV-2, normally just called herpes) cannot be cured, though symptoms can be controlled. Hepatitis B is very easy to pass on during sex, and hepatitis A and C can also be transmitted during certain types of sex. Hepatitis A, B and C can make you ill in the short-term and hepatitis B and C can cause long-term liver disease, which can even be fatal. Hepatitis B and C can make HIV harder to treat.

In some cases people have been reinfected (sometimes also called superinfected) with different or drug-resistant strains of HIV.

Having good sexual health also includes feeling comfortable with your sexuality, and the kinds of sex you are having and who with.

Sexual health check-ups

If you are sexually active, it is wise to have regular sexual health check-ups. These are free and confidential. Many HIV clinics have sexual health clinics (sometimes called GUM clinics) attached, and some HIV clinics now include sexual health screens as part of their routine HIV care. However, you can choose which sexual health clinic you go to.

Most people with HIV in the UK were diagnosed through sexual health clinics, so you may already know what services they provide.

Visits to sexual health clinics normally involve seeing a doctor or nurse who will ask you about the kind of sex you are having, what is wrong and examine you for symptoms. It is important to be honest if you have has unprotected sex so you can have the appropriate tests. Sexual health clinics should be very used to seeing all the communities affected by HIV in the UK, including gay men and Africans, and their services should be non-judgmental.

Check-ups normally involve having swabs taken from the tip of the penis or inside the vagina and from the mouth and throat and anus if you have had oral or anal sex. You will also be asked to provide a urine sample. These are then examined under a microscope or cultured to see if any bacteria grow.

Blood samples are also taken to check for some infections. Some results can be given to you at your visit, but it may be necessary to telephone or come back a week or so later for some other results.

All treatment at NHS sexual health clinics is free of charge and confidential.

If you have a sexually transmitted infection (STI) you may be offered the opportunity to see a health adviser. Health advisers can give you information about STIs and how to avoid them and can help you contact your sexual partners, if this is possible or practical and you agree, so they can be tested and treated. Health advisers can also offer referrals to other specialist services.

Protecting your own and other people's sexual health

Anal and vaginal sex
Unprotected anal and vaginal sex have the greatest risk of HIV transmission. Oral sex is considered in detail in a section below.

The chances of you passing on HIV during unprotected anal or vaginal sex are greatest if you are the active, or insertive partner during sex. The risk is particularly high if you have a high viral load, an untreated STI, or if you ejaculate inside your partner. Similarly, if an HIV-negative person has an untreated STI their chances of contracting HIV from you during unprotected sex are increased.

If you are receptive, or passive during sex, the risk of passing on HIV is reduced, but is still present, especially if you have a high viral load or an untreated STI.

Unprotected vaginal sex also carries the risk of pregnancy. Emergency contraception is available from clinics and from pharmacies without prescription.

Oral sex
The risk of transmitting HIV by oral sex is much less certain.

The Health Protection Agency which monitors HIV in the UK estimates that about 1-3% of all sexual transmission of HIV is due to oral sex.

However the evidence is conflicting, with some doctors and studies suggesting that as many as 8% of HIV infections are due to oral sex, with others putting the figure much lower, even at zero.

The risk from oral sex is much lower than the risk from unprotected anal or vaginal sex. Having a very high viral load, an untreated STI, ejaculating in the mouth of the person sucking and bleeding gums or sores or wounds in the mouth of the person sucking seem to increase the very small risk.

Condoms
Condoms, when used properly, provide excellent protection against getting most STIs and passing on HIV to other people, or being reinfected with another strain of HIV.

In the UK and some other countries it was usual to recommend extra-strong condoms for anal sex, however recent research has found that standard strength condoms are just as safe.

Condoms are usually made of latex. Some people are allergic to latex condoms. If this is the case, then polyurethane condoms are a safe alternative.

A water-based lubricant should be used with condoms, as oil-based ones weaken condoms and can cause tiny tears.

If you are having sex for a long time, then it is safest to change condoms every 30 minutes.

HIV and sexual health clinics provide free condoms, and in some cities free condoms can also be obtained from gay venues. Family planning clinics also provide free condoms.

Condoms should be disposed of as rubbish in a bin and not flushed down the toilet or discarded in the street or in parks or fields.

Use of anti-HIV drugs to prevent infection with HIV

If a person is exposed to HIV during sex, many clinics are willing to provide them with a short-course of anti-HIV drugs to prevent infection. This is called post-exposure prophylaxis, or PEP for short. However, not all clinics offer it for sexual exposure, pointing to worries about side-effects and resistance. Nevertheless, it is becoming more widely available. PEP is not a kind of 'morning after pill' for HIV and it's not 100% effective.

PEP may also be considered in cases of rape and sexual assault where there is a risk of HIV transmission.

It is important to get and take PEP as soon as possible after possible exposure to HIV - ideally within four hours, and certainly within 72 hours, but many believe that this is too late.

If you are taking anti-HIV drugs and have unprotected sex with a person who is HIV-negative or whose HIV status you do not know, or if there is a condom accident during sex you may be tempted to offer them some of your anti-HIV drugs in an attempt to reduce the risk of them becoming infected with HIV. This could involve risks. Some HIV drugs, particularly abacavir (*Ziagen*) and nevirapine (*Viramune*) can cause an allergic reaction or severe side-effects which can be fatal. There is also a chance that the person you are giving your HIV drugs to could already be infected with HIV and taking a few doses of your anti-HIV medicines could lead to resistance developing.

The thought that you may have exposed somebody to the risk of HIV infection is very worrying. If you do think that PEP might be appropriate, go to your local sexual health clinic as soon as possible. If this is closed then go to the accident and emergency department of your local hospital who should contact the on-call HIV doctor.

Undetectable viral load and infectiousness

An undetectable HIV viral load is the goal of anti-HIV treatment. This does not mean that you have been cured of HIV, but that the combination of drugs you are taking has reduced HIV's ability to reproduce so it can no longer be detected in the blood.

An undetectable viral load in blood does not necessarily mean that you are not infectious.

Although many people with undetectable viral loads in their blood also have an undetectable viral load in their sexual fluid and seem less likely to transmit HIV, this is not always the case. Some people with undetectable viral load in their blood have sufficient viral load in their sexual fluids to infect somebody else.

Studies have mainly been conducted in men, and these have found that having an untreated STI, particularly gonorrhoea, increases the chances that HIV viral load will be detectable in semen.

HIV can also be present in cells and it is possible that these could transmit HIV infection even when a person has an undetectable viral load.

In addition, studies have also found that men with high blood viral loads have very high viral loads in their semen and are very infectious.

If a person is resistant to anti-HIV drugs, it is thought they can infect other people with drug resistant HIV, and about 10% of new HIV-infections in the UK are with drug resistant virus. This means that the person newly infected with HIV has limited treatment options before they have taken a single anti-HIV drug.

Reinfection

In addition to STIs, unprotected sex can have other health risks for HIV-positive people. There have been reported cases where a person with HIV has been reinfected, or superinfected with another subtype or strain of HIV which is resistant to anti-HIV drugs.

In some cases this has resulted in the person's HIV viral load increasing and CD4 cell count falling. In addition, their treatment options have been limited because the type of HIV they were reinfected with was resistant to some or all of the anti-HIV drugs they were taking as well as others they had never taken.

It is not known how easy it is for somebody to become reinfected with HIV. So far only a few cases have been reported worldwide, almost all amongst gay men who had unprotected anal sex. However, there has also been a case reported of reinfection involving a heterosexual couple.

Although reinfection appears to be rare, there seem to be some factors that might increase the risk of it happening. Many of the cases occurred soon after a person was first infected with HIV, and others when people were taking a break from anti-HIV treatment.

Further reading

- NAM factsheets, *Candida, Chlamydia, Condoms, Gonorrhoea, Genital warts, Hepatitis B, Hepatitis C, Infectiousness, Herpes, LGV, Mother-to-baby transmission, Oral sex, Post-exposure prophylaxis, Pregnancy and conception, Primary infection, Pubic lice and scabies, Sexual dysfunction, Sperm washing, Syphilis, Sexual health check-ups* and *Unprotected sex.*

- *HIV and hepatitis, HIV and sex* and *HIV and women,* booklets in the information for HIV-positive people series produced by NAM.

- 'HIV transmission,' 'HIV testing,' and 'HIV prevention' in NAM's *HIV AIDS Reference Manual.*

- *Sexually transmitted infections: a guide for people with HIV,* leaflet produced by the Terrence Higgins Trust.

- *Telling People,* produced by the Terrence Higgins Trust.

My experience of anal warts

I've had warts since I was a child - they run in my family. At one point, around the age of 12, I had small warts on most of my fingers. Although I never sought treatment, after a year they suddenly disappeared within the space of a week.

My first bout of genital warts was similarly uneventful. I came home from my first year at university with a self-diagnosis of piles - an unbearable itch in my back passage, and pain and blood after using the toilet. I came away from the GP with an instruction to visit a 'treatment centre' 20 miles away. After being quizzed about my sexual history, an examination revealed the presence of an anal fissure and a single anal wart. The wart was quickly dispatched with a blast of liquid nitrogen.

Eight years later, a couple of years after my HIV diagnosis, the warts on my fingers, plus a few tiny ones on my chin, had returned and been removed with a quick nitrogen zap. When a subsequent examination revealed the presence of a few warts around my back passage, I assumed that a few icy blasts would see them off.

I diligently followed my doctor's advice to pop into the clinic a couple of times a week to have the warts sprayed. I was encouraged by the nurses' reassurances that the warts were small and would soon be gone - especially as my viral load had plummeted from over 120,000 to below 50 copies/ml within a month of starting therapy.

As my bi-weekly visits started to stretch over weeks, then months, a trip back to my doctor revealed that the three months of cryotherapy had achieved nothing, probably on account of my sluggish CD4 count response - rather than climbing obediently, it had continued to fall before hovering around 130 for most of my first year on therapy.

In the two-month wait to be seen by a surgeon, the warts, no longer being kept in check by their regular cold shower or by imiquimod cream, grew to grotesque proportions. One grew inside my anal canal and prolapsed every time I used the toilet, eventually becoming more than 5cm in length and unbelievably painful. I felt disgusting and my sex drive evaporated.

I pinned my hopes on the operation. However, nothing (and no-one) had prepared me for how painful this would turn out to be. After three days in hospital on intravenous antibiotics, there followed eight weeks of a degree of pain I had never imagined. I became terrified of using the toilet, necking laxatives and painkillers in handfuls and teetering on the edge of depression.

To top this off, the warts returned, even stronger, within a month of the surgery. On a return to see the surgeon, he nonchalantly informed me he "would have to repeat the procedure". Gritting my teeth through another three-month delay on a waiting list, the warts became larger than ever: I could barely walk for hours after using the toilet, and I was in tears most days.

Luckily, the second operation was far less traumatic than the first. I was up and ready to leave within hours of coming round, and felt better within days. I only had moderate pain for around a week.

In the two months since the procedure, there is no sign of a recurrence, although the few small warts that couldn't be excised are now enjoying their weekly nitrogen fix. Despite a diagnosis of grade I anal intraepithelial neoplasia (AIN), which is now being monitored in a clinical trial, my mood is climbing almost as quickly as my CD4 count. I'm back on my bike, and finally, after over a year, I'm no longer scared of the toilet.

My hero!
by Philip

Sex. It's messy, fraught with all sorts of psychological problems and yes, it's obviously what got me into this whole predicament in the first place. It is also rather pleasant. I still like to do it, if I am asked; but now, of course, it is a whole different ball game. There are so many risks involved. I mean there were always risks involved before, but now! There is the risk of infecting a negative partner; the risk of acquiring resistance to the drugs you are on or haven't even started; the risk of catching something else that might exacerbate your condition. It's a wonder that I still do it at all, but I soldier valiantly on.

What never really crossed my mind before were the psychological effects of having HIV. It has always been my practice to inform a partner of my status, before we had sex and I had always had encouraging results whenever this had occurred, up until just recently. I don't know quite what has gone wrong with the world over the last year, but I seem to have had several very sobering experiences.

I think the fact that each one seemed to follow on from the other, made it feel more than just a little dispiriting. The first occasion happened several months ago. I had been out at a bar for the evening with friends. Jump forward a few hours and I'm in my bedroom wildly shedding clothes with another guy in anticipation of a night of passion and who knows what else to come.

It suddenly struck me that, unusually for me, I hadn't yet informed him of my status. I broke the news carefully in that cavalier, "it-doesn't-really-matter-because-I-am-always-extremely-safe" kind of way, but suddenly a chill Easterly wind rushed through the room and my friend began to look at me as if I was Old Yeller and it was time to get the rifle.

Giving him points for effort, he did actually go through with the exercise; though speed was obviously a priority for him now. Also, there was one particular thing he was keen to do to me, which he most certainly wasn't going to allow me to to do to him. There were scorch marks on the carpet as he left (within the hour), leaving me feeling considerably less than special.

The next encounter I had didn't even get that far, though once again it occurred in the bedroom. I informed this particular gentleman of my status with a light heart. I should have been more circumspect. Suddenly he was very tired, he had "drunk too much," it was way too late and he had forgotten that he had arranged to meet with a friend for breakfast the next morning. He threw me out and I slunk home feeling like a leper.

Then there was the time I was just told outright: "Sorry, I don't do it with people who have AIDS". I did actually consider telling him that I didn't have AIDS. What I had was HIV, but I felt that the nuance would somehow be lost on him.

Sadly, there are other similar tales from both my own and my friends' experience. I understand why these men have the fears they do, but it is their manners that infuriate me. They lacked finesse, certainly, but principally they lacked respect. It is reasonable of people to be afraid of contracting HIV by having sex with someone who is carrying the virus. They have a choice to make; accidents can happen. No one should ever have sex against their will and I am not saying that either of these men should have gone through with something that frightened them or that they didn't wish to do. However, neither should they have forced me to feel like a pariah.

Should I have remonstrated? Maybe. Maybe not. They had a right to their feelings, but not a right to destroy my self-esteem.

In my negative days, I never treated anyone like that and I had safe sex with a few, some might say 'many', HIV positive men, and never flinched. The sort of behaviour these men display is, I realise now, something at which I cannot continue to be surprised. It is part of the baggage we carry as people with HIV.

Sex is a major part of most of our lives. When we enter into an intimate situation we expose not only our bodies, but part of our souls, and to have that rejected in such a brutal way, creates psychological waves that spread throughout the whole of the rest of our lives. It put me off sex and the possibility of finding a partner for a long time.

We have to be able to lead as normal a life as possible. We are sexual beings and have a right to be treated with the same respect that we give others. Never let anyone try and demean you or make you feel less human for having this disease. Living with it is a struggle, but in many ways that makes us stronger and we in no way contribute less to society either in the office or in the bedroom.

I'd like to leave you on a more upbeat note though, just to show you that not all experiences are like the ones I have described. I think back to a recent, wonderful, though fairly short-lived seven-month affair with a very beautiful Spanish man. Our relationship was serodiscordant (in other words, he was HIV-negative) and yet I was never aware that it ever gave him a moment's concern, other than to make sure that there was always a huge supply of condoms available at any given time in every room in the house.

And let me tell you - that thing that the other guy wouldn't let me do?...He let me do it to him over and over and over again. My hero!

Bored and horny

It's Sunday afternoon and it's raining. I'm bored and horny. However, I've got £20 left over from the night before and this will be enough to buy me entry into a sauna where there should be enough sexy men to relieve more than my boredom.

303

I'm there within half an hour and it's rammed with sexy guys. The trouble is, none seem too interested in me. My self-esteem starts to take a bit of a hammering and I start to wonder what's putting people off. Can people tell I've got HIV just by looking at me? Am I casting off the wrong kind of positive vibe? Or is it that I'm just a bit of a minger? Well, whatever the reason, I persevere and am eventually rewarded. I finally catch somebody's eye. There's no doubting that he's up for it, and rather than fumbling around in the dark he leads me into one of the private cabins and we lock the door.

He very quickly makes it clear what he wants - and it certainly doesn't involve the use of a condom. There's been no discussion of HIV - in all my years of going to saunas there never has been. What's the need anyway? Isn't the use of condoms which are so liberally supplied at saunas are meant to mean to make such discussions unnecessary?

Is he HIV-positive? There's no tell-tale indicators - no evidence of lipodystrophy or a trendy biohazard tattoo to suggest that he's got HIV. Nor do I recognise him as somebody who has 'needs discussion', 'sometimes' or 'never' next to the safer sex option on his gaydar profile. I want to assume he's so HIV-positive so I can comfort myself that, should I give way in the heat of the moment, I wouldn't potentially infect someday with HIV. But then I remember, you're not supposed to assume anything.

There's starting to be a lot of heat in this moment. Yet I'm aware that people have been sent to prison after not telling their sexual partners they have HIV - I don't want to risk my liberty for the sake of an afternoon in a sauna.

The thought of catching something nasty also flashes through my head. An HIV-positive friend recently caught syphilis when he went to a 'bareback' sex party with other HIV-positive men. And in the space of a year I'd picked up chlamydia and gonorrhoea. I'm also aware of reports that some people had been reinfected with strains of drug-resistant HIV after having bareback sex and that there'd been an outbreak of hepatitis C spread by barebacking.

But, on the other hand, I tell myself, he must know the risks. He wants to have unprotected sex in a sauna, dammit! How far should I be held responsible for him? I reassure myself he's probably already HIV-positive. But then, I don't know this, I'm just guessing.

Another thought enters the mix. The knowledge that I'm taking combination therapy and that I have an undetectable viral load is comforting - well, the viral load in my blood was the last time I went to the clinic two months ago. That must surely make a difference, right? And, on top of that - if you'll forgive the pun, I'm the top so my risk of getting reinfected or hep C must be reduced - or at least that's what I tell myself. But, if I'm the top, then my chances of infecting him with HIV are higher if he's negative. I could reduce the risks by so-called 'safer-barebacking' and making sure I don't ejaculate in him, yet, I've heard that even tiny amounts of semen can contain potentially infectious quantities of HIV.

Okay, what do I do? I'm not a saint and I'm horny as hell. I got HIV from having unprotected sex and I know how good it feels, and that's not something I'm going to deny.

But this time things seem so different. On the occasions when I've had unprotected sex since my diagnosis with HIV I've tried to make sure that the other person already had HIV. The internet has made that a lot easier.

I just don't know how to raise the subject now - we're already having sex! I go through the possible options in my head.

It could be that he is too; it could that he isn't or doesn't know and that he couldn't care less; or it could be that he's negative, does care that I'm positive and seem to be about to have unprotected sex with him, goes crazy and hits me for not telling him earlier!

I don't want to create a scene - how British. Nine times out of ten you don't even tell your name to people you meet in a sauna, let alone discuss HIV. Well, perhaps that needs to change, and I may well start changing things now.

Here goes.

The back of my throat is dry when I try to speak - is it nerves or excitement? I croak something inaudible, but it doesn't matter. In the few moments that have passed he's lost interest. He puts his towel around himself, taps me on the shoulder, unlocks the door and leaves the cubicle.

I don't know if I'm relieved or disappointed. And I know that this is unlikely to be the last time I face a situation like this. The problems is, what my mind tells me to do next time and what my dick tells me to do are two completely different things. I'm only human, and I'll do my best to make sure that my mind wins out.

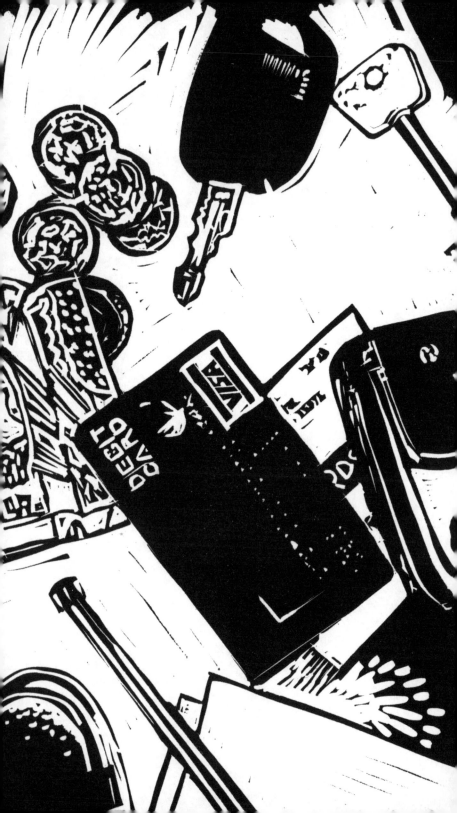

Money

In this chapter you'll find information on

State benefits and rules affecting them,
written by Jackie Brown.

Personal finance issues such as debt,
mortgages and pensions.

Introduction

This chapter provides an introduction to some of the key issues involving money, welfare benefits and personal finance which you might encounter.

Money worries can be a real headache and often get worse if you don't take action, so it's important to tackle them as soon as possible. The information in this section isn't exhaustive, and if you are going to make a claim for welfare benefits, or are thinking of applying for a mortgage, you should seek specialist advice. Regulations governing access to benefits can change very quickly, so, even if you've made a successful application in the past, it's wise to get advice from an accredited benefits adviser. Similarly, some financial advisers have developed a detailed understanding of the financial issues faced by HIV-positive people. A good place to start if you want information on benefits or money advice is the Citizens Advice Bureau. Their website is www.citizensadvice.org.uk and they have branches around the country. All their advice is free.

State benefits

Benefits for people who are too ill to work

This section was written in early 2006. Rules regarding state benefits are continually changing. If you have any questions about state benefits you would be well advised to seek specialist advice. THT Direct is the signposting and telephone advice section of Terrence Higgins Trust. They can be contacted on 0845 1221200. If you have a benefit or debt problem, they can give you advice, and if necessary details of agencies in your area who are able to assist with your problem. They can also refer to THT's Specialist Advice Centre if appropriate

If you are unfit to work, your doctor will give you a medical certificate, to enable you to claim benefits.

If you are employed, you may be entitled to Statutory Sick Pay. You must normally earn at least £82 per week (£84 from April 2006). A certificate is not necessary for the first week, but is necessary thereafter.

If you do not have a job, or have not been able to work for more than six months due to ill health, you should claim Incapacity Benefit. As well as being unfit to work you have to have paid national insurance contributions in order to get incapacity benefit. A medical certificate is necessary, unless you have received a letter from the DWP stating that there is no need for you to send in further certificates.

The test for incapacity benefit is the Personal Capability Assessment, usually payment is made for the first six months of the claim, and then a form called an IB50 is sent to you, asking you to assess whether you can do a series of tests. Often this form is followed up by a request for you to see a Department of Work and Pensions (DWP) doctor, to see if s/he agrees with your self assessment. This often leads to withdrawal of benefit.

However, some groups of people are exempt from this test. Amongst people with HIV there are two main groups who are exempt, the first, which affects all claimants, is people who get the highest rate of care component of Disability Living Allowance (DLA).

There is also an exempt group specific to people with HIV. This is where there are tumours or opportunistic infections as a result of your HIV diagnosis. If this is the case for you, it is worth asking your doctor to state that you have the tumour/opportunistic infection on your medical certificate, which is likely to lead to exemption from the test, and may stop loss of benefits.

If you are under 20, it is possible to claim incapacity benefit without fulfilling the national insurance contributions, this is known as Non Contributory Incapacity Benefit. If you are a student, it may be possible to claim up to the age of 25.

When you claim incapacity benefit, you should also make a claim for Income Support. Some people will not be entitled to incapacity benefit because they have not paid enough contributions, however, it is necessary to claim incapacity benefit as well as income support, so that the DWP will note that you are unfit to work, and will pay income support to you whilst you are sick, if you fulfil all the other relevant criteria.

Income Support is a means tested benefit, which means that the DWP will ask if you have any money coming in, and if it is over the amount which is allowed each week (known as the applicable amount), you will not get income support. It is common for people to get a reduced amount of income support, particularly if they are getting other benefits, such as child benefit or incapacity benefit. They will also ask whether you have any capital, if you up to £3000, it will be ignored, if you have between £3000 and £8000, income support will be paid at a reduced rate, if you have over £8,000, you have more than the 'capital limit' and income support will not be paid. (If this is the case, don't forget to reapply if your capital falls below the capital limit, however the DWP may still refuse benefit if they decide that you have deprived yourself of capital in order to obtain benefits). The figures above are the same for a couple as for a single person.

When you claim income support, the claim pack will also include claims for Housing Benefit and Council Tax Benefit. Housing benefit is payable if you rent your property and your income is low. If you own your property you should ask for Housing Costs, which will not be paid at first, but if you are long term sick, you may get some help with your mortgage interest payments.

If you are not claiming Housing and/or Council Tax Benefits at the same time as income support, you can get claim packs from your local authority, which will have a department dedicated to these benefits.

These benefits are also means tested, the rules are much the same as for income support, but the capital limit for Housing and Council Tax benefit is £16,000, so it is possible to be refused income support because your savings are too high, but still get housing and council tax benefit.

Some people get a benefit called Severe Disablement Allowance, it is no longer possible to put in a fresh claim for this, but it is paid to people who have not paid national insurance contributions, and have been sick for some time. Usually this applies to people who have never worked due to disability. Non-contributory incapacity benefit (above) is the newer equivalent.

If you have been sick for over a year, and getting one of the sickness related benefits above, your income support will increase, as you will be awarded a disability premium. This will not happen if you have been getting DLA, as the premium will apply from the date DLA is awarded, if you have a claim for income support.

Disability Living Allowance (DLA)
Disability Living Allowance (DLA) is payable when there are care or mobility needs. The form for this is long, and the questions can be difficult to answer. Wherever possible get an advisor to help with completion of the form, as many appeals arise simply because there is not enough information in the form.

If you do have to fill in the form yourself, just remember to address any difficulties you have with walking or looking after yourself. (For example, many people with HIV have night sweats. They wake up wet and uncomfortable. If it is difficult for you to change the bed, perhaps because of fatigue, dizziness, peripheral neuropathy or whatever give details. If you don't change a wet bed because you feel too unwell, tell them. Say what makes it difficult, and what help you need. If you live alone and just have to get on with things, give details of the help you would need if there was a carer there to look after you).

The care component is paid at three rates:

- Highest - for people who need attention and/or supervision both day and night.

- Middle - for people who need attention and/or supervision during the day or the night.

- Lower - for people who need attention for a significant portion of the day (classed as an hour or more, but not for most of the day), or who cannot cook a meal for one person if they had the ingredients and facilities.

A grant of the highest rate of care component of DLA entitles you to the Enhanced Disability Premium on your income support. It also means that you are exempt from the Personal Capability Assessment - the test for incapacity benefit.

A grant of the middle or highest rate of care component gives rise to Severe Disability Premium on your income support, if you do not have any adults living in your home who are not financially dependent on you (and part of your benefit claim) and if nobody is claiming carers allowance for you.

A grant of any rate of care or mobility component of DLA gives rise to the Disability premium on income support.

The mobility component of DLA is paid at two rates:

Higher rate - for people who either cannot walk at all, or cannot walk without severe discomfort - usually the benchmark is around 50 yards, and severe discomfort can be pain, breathlessness, fatigue, anything which makes it difficult for you to walk.

If you get the higher rate of mobility component, you may be able to get a motability car - leased car from a company which takes the mobility component of DLA as payment for the lease of the vehicle. The telephone number for Motability is 0845 456 4566.

Also, if you get higher rate of mobility component, you or your carer can be exempt from paying car tax on a car used just by you or for you. You can get an exemption form, and/or claim pack for DLA by phoning the Disability Benefits Centre on 08457 123456.

You can also contact your local authority for details of disabled parking and travel permits for the disabled.

Lower rate - for people who need supervision when they go to unfamiliar places. Most commonly this is for people who experience panic attacks when they have to go somewhere new.

If your doctor believes that it is not unexpected that you will die within the next six months, you can make a claim under the Special Rules. Your doctor will have to complete a form called a DS1500, giving reasons for his opinion. Special rules cases are fast tracked, and you should have a decision within a couple of weeks. During this time, the evidence of your doctor will be examined by a DWP doctor. If the DWP doctor agrees with your doctor's assessment you will automatically be awarded the highest rate of care component. If you have mobility problems, you will have to complete the part of the claim pack that deals with mobility.

If you are over 65, you should claim Attendance Allowance, rather than DLA. Attendance Allowance is only paid at two rates, lower, which is the equivalent of middle rate of care component of DLA, with the same criteria, and higher, which is the equivalent of the highest rate of DLA care component. There is no mobility component of attendance allowance, however if you have an award of mobility component of DLA when you reach your 65th birthday, payment will continue until the award runs out, or until the DWP look again at your award.

Neither DLA nor Attendance Allowance is taxable.

Benefits for carers
If you care for a person who gets DLA at the middle or higher rate of care component for 35 hours a week or more, then you may be eligible for Carer's

Allowance. It is best to take advice before applying for carers allowance, particularly if the person you are caring for is your partner, when you may actually lose money by making the application if you are in receipt of income support as a couple.

However, if you live alone, and apply for Carer's Allowance, it can be topped up with Income Support.

Benefits for people who are unemployed

Contribution-Based Job Seeker's Allowance is payable for six months, assuming you meet the contribution conditions. It does not matter how much savings you have and how much other money is coming into the home.

Income-Based Job Seeker's Allowance is payable either when insufficient national insurance contributions have been paid, or at the end of the six month period. It has the same income and capital restrictions as income support. It also passports to Housing and Council Tax Benefits in the same way. As with Income Support, you can claim for an adult dependent, but if you are responsible for children, you should claim Child Tax Credit.

In order to get Job Seeker's Allowance it is necessary to sign on as available for work, and to be actively seeking employment.

Benefits for people in work

It is possible to get DLA whilst working, most commonly people will get the middle rate of care component for night time care needs, and sometimes mobility component too.

If you are working less than 16 hours a week you may be entitled to Income Support. However, if your partner is working this is unlikely, as the income of both of you will be taken into consideration too.

Working Tax Credit: Is a top up benefit, administered by the Inland Revenue. You need to work full time - defined as over 16 hours a week (or in the case of a couple, one of you needs to be in full time employment).

Extra payments can be made if you have a physical or mental disability which puts you at a disadvantage when seeking work.

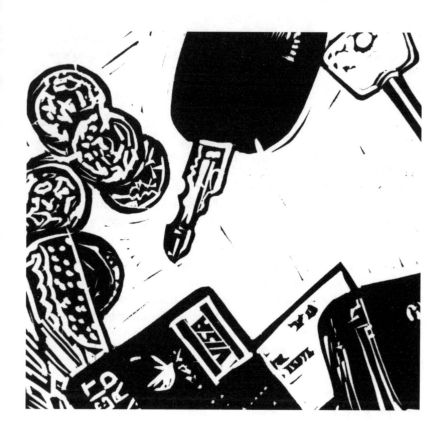

If you have childcare costs associated with your work, you may be entitled to the childcare element of Working Tax Credit.

Housing and Council Tax Benefit may also be payable if your income is low.

Benefits if you are pregnant
Statutory Maternity Pay is payable if you are employed. It is payable for a total of 26 weeks, and cannot start before the 11th week before the date your baby is due, although you can defer it to start later.

You will receive 90% of your average weekly earnings for the first six weeks. For the remaining 20 weeks you will receive 90% of your average weekly earnings, or £106 per week, whichever is less. It is important to write to your local Revenue National Insurance Contributions Office to claim national insurance credits whilst you are off of work. Your employer should have the address.

Statutory Maternity Allowance is payable if you have worked but are no longer working. You need to have worked for at least 26 weeks in the 66 weeks before your baby is due, and to have earned at least £30 a week during that period. As with SMP, you cannot claim before the 11th week before the baby is due, and it is paid at £106 per week.

Benefits if you are looking after children

Child Benefit - until the child is 16, or if s/he remains in full time non-advanced (not degree level) education, until s/he is 19.

Child Tax Credit - payable to people responsible for a child. It is possible to get child tax credit even if you are part of a couple where both work, as long as your joint annual income is below £50,000.

If you are working and on a low income, child tax credit may be available.

If you are a single parent, who is not working, you can claim Income Support for yourself and Child Tax Credit for your children.

If you are on income based job seekers allowance, and have children, then you can claim child tax credit for them.

Income Support some people are still getting income support for their children. Their numbers are diminishing, as the aim of the government is to take away the income support payment for children, and replace it with child tax credits.

Housing and Council Tax Benefits may be available.

You may be entitled to free school dinners for your children. Also free prescriptions, eye tests and dentistry are available.

Benefits if you are retired

Pension Credit is essentially income support for the retired, and carries the same passports to Housing and Council Tax Benefits.

State Retirement Pension Extra pension is available to those who have paid national insurance contributions and their widows.

Benefits for students

Generally speaking, students cannot get means tested benefits, however if you are in receipt of Incapacity Benefit, Income Support as sick, Severe Disablement Allowance, or DLA you will be deemed to be a disabled student, and as such may have an entitlement to benefit.

Please be aware that your student grants and loans will affect the amount you get, and if possible seek benefit advice before making the decision to study.

Civil partnerships and benefits

Since the Civil Partnership Bill came into effect on 5th December 2005, same sex couples are treated in the same way as heterosexual couples for benefits purposes. Registered civil partners are treated in the same way as married couples, and unregistered civil partners are treated as co-habitees. The main difference between the treatment of married/registered and unmarried/unregistered couples for benefits purposes is that married/registered couples can access death benefits and pensions in respect of their partners. However, as with all benefits, the rules are complex, and if in doubt, seek advice.

Benefits for asylum seekers and those with no leave to enter/remain in the UK

Generally speaking, this group has no right to benefits. Although there may be some exceptions. Asylum seekers who applied before 1996 and still have not had a decision on their immigration application, and those who applied before 2000 and have not had a decision should seek advice.

Also, the restriction is on 'public funds' which are defined by legislation. The rule of thumb is that benefits which rely on contributions, such as incapacity benefit, contribution based job seekers allowance and statutory maternity pay are not public funds, and therefore if you have worked you may be able to claim these if you have paid enough national insurance contributions. Seek advice before claiming.

Public Fund restriction: You may have leave to enter/remain in the UK subject to a restriction which says that you have no recourse to public funds. Do not claim benefits without taking advice on whether the relevant benefit is a public fund. If you make a claim for a benefit which is a public fund, it is a criminal offence. In reality, what happens is that they do not press charges, but when you apply for your leave to be extended, it is refused.

'Mixed' couples: Sometimes one member of a couple has an entitlement to benefit, but their spouse/partner does not. Generally speaking, the partner with recourse to public funds can claim benefit, but it will not include an amount for their partner.

However, in a couple where there is a child who does not have leave to remain, and a parent who does, the parent can claim child benefit and child tax credit in respect of that child.

Once you receive leave to remain without restrictions you are entitled to benefits in the same way as everyone else. If you have been given refugee status (granted asylum) it is currently possible to claim income support back to the date when you first claimed asylum. However this is due to change at some stage - the date has yet to be announced, and a loan offered to refugees, subject to their ability to repay. It is vital that you make the application for backdated income support within 28 days of the date of the letter from the Home Office confirming your refugee status; otherwise you will lose the backdated money.

Unfortunately, it is a common experience for people who have just been granted leave to have a difficult time when they first go to claim benefits, delays in issuing national insurance numbers, and because of that delays in payment of benefits, are commonplace. If you have this experience, please seek advice.

If your application for benefits is turned down always seek advice. Most decisions are open to appeal, and it is wise to seek professional advice on whether you have any grounds for appeal.

Be aware of the deadlines, most benefits give one month from the date of decision, but Housing and Council Tax Benefit give only 28 days. Both of these periods can be extended by two weeks by asking for written reasons for the decision, always do this if you cannot get an appointment with an adviser within the deadlines.

If you do successfully appeal a benefit decision, then benefit is paid back to the date of claim.

Debt management

Organisations which provide benefits advice and information are often able to help you to work out how to manage any debts which you may have.

An advisor will look at your financial commitments and income with you. They'll prioritise your financial commitments and debts, giving the highest priority to your rent or mortgage, utility bills, council tax, and any fines which you may have. If you have any money left over, then a repayment scheme for credit cards, loans and other debts can be worked out. If you are very badly in debt, they will be able to advice you on bankruptcy or administration.

Even if you feel able to manage your own financial affairs, don't ignore letters from banks or credit card companies. Debts won't go away unless you do something about them, and will become more of a headache the longer you leave them.

The Social Fund

Covers a whole series of benefits, which are briefly described below.

Community Care Grants: Designed to keep or establish people in the community, particularly applicable if you have just come out of prison, hospital or temporary accommodation. Also applies to help alleviate exceptional pressures on a family, and to meet travel costs within the UK to visit someone who is ill, attend a relative's funeral, ease domestic crisis, visit child pending residence hearing, or move to suitable accommodation.

It is necessary to be in receipt of income support, income based Job Seeker's Allowance or Pension Credit when you make the application. As a grant, it is not repayable.

Budgeting Loans: Aimed to help with the major expenses which everyone has periodically, such as replacing household items. It is a better alternative than credit, as there is no interest, however the amount you can get will depend on the amount the DWP deems you can repay.

As with the Community Care Grant, it is necessary to be in receipt of income support, income based Job Seeker's Allowance or Pension Credit when you make your application. As a loan, it will be recovered directly from your means tested benefit.

If you are not sure whether a grant or a loan is applicable, always apply for a grant, the decision maker will consider a loan if the grant cannot be paid.

Crisis Loans: For immediate, short term crisis. Not necessary to be in receipt of benefits, but it is necessary to be able to show that you can repay the loan. It can never be over £1,000.

The Regulated Social Fund

Sure Start Maternity Grants: £500 for each child or expected child. You or your partner need to be getting Income Support, income based job seekers allowance, child tax credit at a rate that exceeds the family element or working tax credit with disability or severe disability element.

The form SF100 is available from job centre plus or DWP website. As with other maternity based benefits, you can claim from eleven weeks before the baby is due, but unlike other benefits, the initial claim can be up to three months from the date of confinement.

Funeral payments: You need to be in receipt of a means tested benefit - includes housing and council tax benefit to apply. You need to be responsible for the cost of the funeral and either partner, parent, offspring or close friend or relative of the person who has died.

This does not cover the whole cost of the funeral, please ensure that you seek advice before committing yourself to paying for an expensive funeral which you may not be able to afford.

Winter fuel payments: if you are over 60, and are getting means tested benefits. The amount you get depends upon your age, £200 if aged 60-69, £250 if aged 70-79 and £300 if 80 plus. Not everyone needs to claim, seek advice if you are in these age groups.

Cold weather payments: Paid only where the weather is below freezing for a whole week. You need to be in receipt of pension credit, or income support/income based Job Seeker's Allowance which includes a disability or pensioner premium, or be responsible for a child under five.

Personal finance

It's an indication of how much the outlook for HIV-positive people has improved since effective treatment became available that this book includes a section providing information on mortgages and pensions - something that was lacking in the 1996 publication, *Living with HIV and AIDS*.

Mortgages

Getting a mortgage is not actually any harder if you are HIV-positive. Mortgage lenders don't usually ask any questions about your health or HIV status. All they're interested in is seeing that you meet the financial criteria for the mortgage you are applying for.

However, there can still be problems. You may well be asked to take out life assurance to cover the mortgage in the event of your death. Even though the prognosis for many people with HIV has improved dramatically recently there's still no life assurance policy which will provide cover for people with HIV. Don't lie about your health to get life assurance cover. A better plan might be to find a mortgage lender that doesn't require life assurance.

It's also likely to be impossible for you to obtain heath insurance to cover your mortgage payments in the event of you becoming too ill to work. Again, don't lie. Your claim won't be successful and you'll just be wasting money on premiums.

Pensions

Having HIV will not be a problem if you are thinking of joining a company pension scheme or starting a personal pension plan. However, you might ask, why bother? Improving treatment for HIV could well mean that you live to pension age and beyond. What's more, if you were to become ill, or even die before retirement age, the terms of your pension could mean that you still get benefits from it, such as a medical retirement pension or, in the event of your death, a payment to your partner (husband or wife, registered Civil Partner or specifically nominated partner who you are not in a formal, legal relationship with) or next-of-kin.

It's worth getting specialist financial advice, and some financial advisers have a lot of experience of working with HIV-positive clients. Similar advice might also be available from your local HIV support organisation.

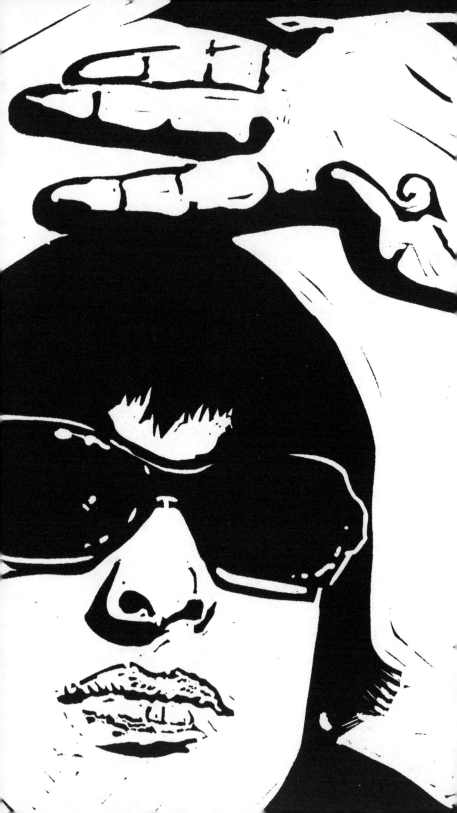

Travel

In this chapter you'll find information on

Entry restrictions that some countries
impose on people with HIV.

Travelling with your HIV medication.

Your health and travel.

Health insurance for people with HIV and
how to obtain medical care abroad.

Travel vaccinations.

A caution not to take a break from
HIV treatment to travel unless you
have discussed the safety of this with
your doctor.

There is a testimony from an HIV-positive
women about her experiences of travel.

Introduction

Being HIV-positive can mean that you need to make detailed plans before travelling. This section provides some general information on how to find out whether a country puts restrictions on entry for people with HIV, and if so, how to deal with these, as well as on travel insurance, vaccinations and receiving medical treatment away from home.

Entry restrictions

Find out if a country you are planning to visit has any entry restrictions for people with HIV. It's generally well known that you cannot visit the USA if you are HIV-positive except in very special circumstances. But other countries also place restrictions on either temporary or long-term visits by individuals with HIV.

The most reliable way of finding out if a country you want to visit restricts entry by people with HIV is to call the embassy or consulate. If you do this, you should not reveal your name or the fact that you are HIV-positive to them. An HIV advocacy or support agency might be willing to do this for you. You might also consider contacting an HIV service organisation in the country you are thinking of travelling to and enquire about entry restrictions. NAM's *HIV & AIDS Services Worldwide* provides listings of major HIV organisations with contact details.

If a country you want to travel to does have entry restrictions, then you need to decide if you want to take the risk of travelling. If you look ill, or are a gay man or an African, you might be more likely to be stopped by customs or immigration, and if they establish that you are HIV-positive, they will probably refuse entry and deport you. Similarly, if you have haemophilia and are travelling with clotting factors or injecting equipment, it's likely that customs officers will question you about your HIV status.

If you are a citizen of an EU country, or have the right to live in an EU country, then there should be no restrictions on your admittance to another EU member state. But because you receive free HIV care in the UK doesn't necessarily mean that you will be entitled to it in the country you are visiting.

If you are planning a long-term visit or permanent move to another country, make sure at a very early stage in your planning that your HIV status isn't going to be a problem. A good place to start would be to contact an HIV service organisation in the country you want to move to. NAM's *AIDS Organisations Worldwide* and *European AIDS Directory* list major organisations that you might want to consider contacting.

Countries and their entry restrictions

Detailed below is information on individual countries' policies regarding entry for people with HIV:

Albania
No restrictions.

Algeria
Citizens returning from work abroad and members of the armed forces will be required to take an HIV test.

Angola
All nationalities require a visa to enter Angola.

A negative HIV status certificate is required to obtain a residence visa to work. Ordinary, transit and residential visas do not require this.

Anguilla
For British nationals there are no restrictions although there are reports of entry being refused to other foreign nationals suspected of having, or known to have, HIV.

Argentina
No restrictions on visits of less than three months. No distinction between applicants from different countries. The usual documentation is required for longer visits and residence applications. However, HIV screening is included in the health control

of immigrants. Foreigners suffering from diseases that reduce their ability to work will not be admitted on a temporary or permanent residence permit.

Armenia
Entry prohibited for HIV-positive people. Also, people who fall ill during their stay in the country may be deported, although the actual legislation on this matter is still being prepared.

Aruba
HIV testing is required for intending immigrants.

Australia
Everyone except those with Australian or New Zealand passports must have a visa. For short business or tourism visits, travellers must sign a declaration of good health. Those who are unable to sign must provide details of any health problems. It is unlikely that those with HIV will be denied entry for short visits, but each case is considered on its merits.

HIV tests are required for foreigners who want to immigrate permanently to Australia.

Anyone working in food handling, or in a classroom situation will be required to have a medical. This is largely to prevent the spread of tuberculosis.

For stays over one year in duration, a medical with chest X-ray and blood test is required. All cases are considered on their merits.

In general, HIV-positive status is not a problem unless there is a public health risk (i.e. tuberculosis) or considerable expense by the health service is involved, or access to limited treatment resources for Australians may be reduced.

Austria
There appear to be no entry restrictions as such although the city of Klagenfurt requires persons applying for a residence permit to be certified as HIV-negative. Health certificate is required with application for a residence permit for more and six months from non-EU citizens.

Azerbaijan
No known restrictions.

Bahamas
The Ministry of Health have recommended that HIV-positive people should not be allowed to enter the country.

Bahrain
No restrictions on stays of less than four weeks. No questions are asked - but if a person were to declare their HIV-positive status they would be refused entry. There are exceptions for diplomatic staff.

Individuals will not be permitted employment in food handling or patient/child care if they are HIV-positive.

Bangladesh
There are no specific entry regulations for people with HIV, and this also applies to long-term residence. If is possible, however, that foreigners with HIVare deported if the competent authorities find out about their condition.

Barbados
At present, no restrictions for holiday trips. A medical is required for a long-term stay, or for a work permit, and it is thought unlikely that an HIV-positive person would be allowed into the country on a long-term basis.

Belarus
All persons staying longer than three months must produce evidence of their HIV status.

Belgium
All non-European Community nationals intending to study or undertake work permit employment must undergo an HIV test by a Belgian-approved doctor in their country of origin. No visas are granted for people who test HIV-positive.

Belize
Foreign nationals applying for citizenship must produce a negative HIV test certificate on arrival issued not more than two months earlier.

Benin
No restrictions for short-time tourist stays. HIV testing required for longer-term stays.

Bolivia
No regulations for short tourism or business visits - but compulsory Yellow Fever Vaccine for all visitors. This live vaccine is not recommended for those with compromised immunity.

A medical with blood test is required for short- or long-term residency applications.

Anyone staying more than 90 days and applicants for work permits will be required to provide evidence of their HIV status.

Bosnia-Herzegovina
No entry res1trictions for HIV-positive people, However foreigners applying for a permanent residence must present a negative HIV test result.

Botswana
HIV testing required from students beginning their studies.

Brazil
There are no entry restrictions for people living with HIV.

Brunei
No mandatory testing for short-term tourist stays. However, people known to be HIV-positive are prohibited from entering, and expulsed if HIV infection is detected. Doctors have a duty to immediately inform authorities.

Bulgaria
Foreign nationals intending to stay for 30 days or longer are tested within 72 hours of arrival. The test is also required from Bulgarian nationals who have been abroad for longer than 30 days.

Burkina Faso
There are no entry restrictions for HIV-positive persons. However, in order to obtain an entry visa, foreigners must be vaccinated against yellow fever, a live vaccine which is not recommended for those with compromised immunity.

Burundi
No restrictions for HIV-positive people.

Cambodia
Though a foreigner can be expelled if he/she poses a threat to national security, health is not mentioned as grounds for expulsion.

Cameroon
There are no restrictions on entry and residence entitlement relating to public health.

Canada
People entering Canada for short tourist stays or temporary residents for less than six months are nor required to disclose their HIV status or to be tested.

Mandatory HIV testing of all prospective immigrants occurs. However, a recent (June 2001) policy change means that the status of would-be immigrants who test

HIV-positive will be decided on a case by case basis. People found to be HIV-positive will not be automatically excluded.

UK passport holders can travel to Canada without the need for a visa.

Chile
There are no specific restrictions for those wishing to travel to Chile. A medical certificate is needed for those applying for a work permit or residency. Foreign students are also tested for HIV. If a person is found to be HIV-positive he or she will be denied entry.

China
Foreign nationals applying for residence or intending to stay more than six months must have an HIV test certificate approved by a Chinese Embassy or consulate, or undergo a test in China within 20 days of arrival. It is reported that random testing at the point of entry is now unofficial Chinese policy. Entry is denied and deportation is likely for foreigners who are found to be HIV-positive. Testing is not required for entry or residency in Hong Kong.

Colombia
A medical certificate is required for those who are applying for a long stay visa, work permit or residency. Anyone who is suspected of being HIV-positive will not be admitted for short visits.

Costa Rica
People wishing to work or live in Costa Rica are requested to present a medical certificate. There is no specification regarding HIV status.

Cote d'Ivoire (Ivory Coast)
No restrictions for HIV-positive individuals.

Croatia
No restrictions.

Cuba
Foreign students, foreign workers and long-term foreign residents are screened for

HIV; people found to be HIV-positive are reportedly repatriated.

Cyprus
All foreign workers and students are required to undergo medical examinations, including an AIDS test. Under immigration laws, any carriers of contagious and infectious diseases, including HIV, are considered illegal immigrants and permission of entry is at the discretion of the Minister of the Interior.

Czech Republic
No restrictions.

Denmark
No restrictions.

Dominican Republic
A negative HIV test certificate is required for a work permit or application for permanent residency.

Ecuador
Those applying for a long-term residency are normally requested to test for HIV.

Egypt
All foreigners intending to stay in the country for three months or more must have an HIV test on arrival. Spouses of Egyptian nationals are exempt. Foreigners requiring work permits must be tested but their spouses are exempt. No residence or work permit will be granted if test result is positive.

Foreign defence contractors at Egyptian military establishments must produce an HIV test certificate.

Eritrea
No restrictions.

Estonia
No restrictions on entry for HIV-positive individuals unless applying for a work permit or residence.

Ethiopia
No restrictions.

Fiji
People with HIV/AIDS are not allowed to enter the Fiji Islands.

Finland
No restrictions. However, according to a clause in the Finnish law persons who "knowingly transmit" HIV may be deported.

Gabon
All travellers require a medical certificate to enter the country. No specific HIV restrictions apply.

Georgia
All foreigners staying longer than one month are required to provide evidence of their HIV status, provided that the test certification was issued at least 30 days before arrival.

Germany
Foreign nationals applying for residence in Bavaria and tourists staying more than four months must undergo an HIV test. Certain nationalities are exempt.

Ghana
No restrictions.

Greece
Non-EU foreign students and foreigners wishing to work in Greece are required to take an HIV test, as are women intending to work in 'entertainment centres'.

Guatemala
No restrictions.

Guinea
No restrictions.

Guyana
All foreigners staying longer than three months are required to provide evidence of their HIV status. However the restrictions may be lifted in the near future.

Haiti
No restrictions.

Honduras
A medical certificate is part of the visa requirement for those wishing to travel or work in Honduras.

Hong Kong
Intending immigrants must undergo HIV-testing.

Hungary
No restrictions for short-term tourist stays. No HIV testing on entry. An HIV test is required for anyone who wants to stay in the country for more than one year. Additionally, some employers may require their staff to undergo HIV testing.

All students over 18, anyone between the ages of 18 and 70 with a visa valid for at least one year and anyone extending a stay to a year or more must provide evidence of their HIV status. Accredited journalists and diplomats are excluded from this requirement.

Iceland
In general, neither a medical certificate nor an HIV test result is required when entering Iceland. Immigration authorities require foreign nationals to perform a health exam when applying for a residence permit. If an infectious disease (i.e. tuberculosis or AIDS) is discovered, the person immediately enters the Icelandic health care system. The general rule, which states that a foreigner has to have been staying in the country for at least six months before he can join the local public health system, is not applied in this case.

India
No restrictions for short-term tourist stays. HIV testing required for anyone wishing to stay in India longer than one year. There are also specific regulations, which apply to all foreign students admitted to an Indian university. People with a known HIV infection are not granted visas.

Indonesia
There are no specific entry or residence regulations for people with HIV/AIDS. Neither a medical certificate nor an HIV test result is required when entering the country. Foreigners with a known HIV infection are not subject to specific residence regulations. There are no regulations regarding the control, deportation or expulsion of those concerned.

Iran
Foreign nationals intending to work in Iran or to stay for more than three months must produce an HIV test certificate.

Iraq
People with HIV are not allowed to enter Iraq. A very recent test result has to be presented on entry, or else the test is performed on the spot. Those concerned are immediately expelled.

Exceptions: Holders of diplomatic passports or service passports while on official duty. People officially invited by the government and staying for 15 days or less. People older than 65. Children under age 12, who are in possession of a declaration from their parents, which states that they are not haemophiliacs and have never received a blood transfusion.

Ireland (The Republic of)
There are no specific entry or residence regulations for people with HIV.

Israel
There are no specific entry regulations for people with HIV travelling to Israel. The only condition is that they must have health insurance.

People intending to stay more than three months to work or study are required to show a medical certificate which includes information on HIV status.

Italy
No restrictions for people with HIV.

Jamaica
No restrictions for people with HIV.

Japan
There are no restrictions for people with HIV who wish to travel or work in Japan.

Jordan
For a stay of more than 30 days, a medical examination by a Health Ministry laboratory is obligatory. In the case of positive test result, the applicant has to leave the country at very short notice.

Kazakhstan
A negative test result has to be provided when applying for a work or residence permit. It is recommended to carry a certified copy of a test result certificate in Russian language. This way it can be avoided to undergo an HIV test in Kazakhstan, a procedure that, in some cases, has to be repeated every three months.

Kenya
Foreigners may be excluded for refusing to undergo a medical examination. Though no entry restrictions have been specifically adopted relating to HIV.

Korea (Democratic People's Republic)
There is no legal provision regarding the entry of people with HIV. Not everybody is requested to present a medical certificate or a specific document of an AIDS examination when entering the country. However, if a person's HIV-positive status becomes known, he/she is sent back to his/her country of origin. The reason given for this is the lack of experience with HIV and the lack of treatment options.

Korea (South)
People with HIV are not permitted to enter the country. However, for a stay of up to three months, it is not mandatory to prove one's HIV status (for those visitors who do not require a visa). There are controls at the border regarding the HIV status. If a person's HIV-positive status becomes known, he/she is expelled.

Kuwait
No HIV testing is required for visitors or business travellers. The visa application for a long-term stay requires a doctor's certificate. In the case of an HIV infection, no visa is granted.

Kyrgyzstan
All foreigners excluding diplomats staying more than one month are required to provide evidence of their HIV status.

Laos
There are no specific entry or residence regulations for people with HIV.

Latvia
No HIV testing on entry, but anyone seeking a residency permit has to present a test result.

Lebanon
Anyone planning to work in Lebanon must undergo an HIV test.

Lesotho
It is at the discretion of the border police as to whether or not a person may enter into Lesotho. However, no medical checks are carried out.

Libya
No restrictions for short stays, but HIV testing is obligatory for longer stays requiring a residence permit. In the case of a proven HIV infection, foreign nationals are required to leave the country immediately, or are not allowed to enter in the first place.

Lithuania
Applicants for permanent residence permits.

Luxemburg
No specific regulations regarding the entry of people with HIV, although Luxemburg law stipulates that entry can be denied on health grounds.

Macedonia
No restrictions.

Madagascar
No restrictions.

Malawi
No entry restrictions. A health certificate is not required for longer stays and applications for residence permits either.

Malaysia
HIV testing for foreign nationals who apply for a work permit for unskilled labour.

Special provisions for domestic staff and construction workers from developing countries (Bangladesh, Pakistan, Indonesia, the Philippines); denial of permission to enter, or expulsion, if the HIV test result is positive.

Maldives
Long-term visitors are required to undergo an HIV test in the Maldive Islands.

Mali
There are no entry restrictions for HIV-positive persons. However, yellow fever vaccination is required. This is not recommended in immune compromised individuals.

Malta
No restrictions.

Marshall Islands
Temporary visitors staying more than thirty days and applicants for residence and work permits are required to produce evidence of HIV status.

Mauritius
HIV test required for foreign nationals who want to work in Mauritius or who apply for permanent residence.

Mexico
Foreigners with a known HIV infection are not subject to specific entry or residence regulations. The deportation of an HIV-positive person is only possible in the case of a very severe offence.

Micronesia
Anyone staying over 90 days and anyone holding a work permit is required to undergo an HIV test.

Monaco
No restrictions.

Moldavia
Foreign nationals who are HIV positive are not allowed to enter Moldavia. A medical certificate is required on entry, although tourists are exempt. In addition, foreign tourists need to pass a health exam conducted by the Moldavian Health Authorities. Such a certificate is also necessary if a foreign national wishes to get married in Moldavia. HIV testing is required of anybody wishing to stay longer than three months.

Mongolia
A test result is requested on entry. However, this law is apparently not applied. Foreign students must have an HIV test on arrival, repeated several months later. Foreigners staying longer than 30 days may also be required to undergo testing, though this is not an official law and is only selectively applied.

Montserrat
Foreign nationals, including university students who are applying for or renewing work or residence must produce a negative HIV certificate.

Morocco
No restrictions.

Mozambique
No restrictions.

Namibia
No restrictions.

Nepal
No restrictions. However some foreign visitors with HIV have reportedly been deported.

Netherlands
No restrictions.

New Zealand
No restrictions for stays of up to twelve months.

From early 2005, New Zealand started undertaking HIV screening for migrants. The full set of changes, including screening for HIV, and a wider and updated set of tests for other expensive-to-treat conditions, was implemented for people seeking to be in New Zealand for longer than twelve months.

Nicaragua
No restrictions for short-term stays. For stays of more than three months, the residence permit has to be extended by the immigration authorities. In this case, the presentation of a medical certificate is requested.

Extended residency will only exceptionally be granted to HIV-positive people.

Nigeria
Immigration officers may refuse entry to any foreigners who are undesirable for medical reasons. Also, immigration officers may refuse entry to any foreigners living with HIV, whose home country would apply restrictions to Nigerian nationals.

Norway
Persons who stay in Norway for longer than three months are offered a voluntary tuberculosis test and an HIV test, in order to arrange for any necessary treatment as quickly as possible.

Myanmar (Burma)
No restrictions.

Oman
There is no clear information on whether or not HIV testing is required for tourists.

Persons whose HIV-positive status becomes known are immediately deported.

Compulsory testing on entry for foreign nationals wishing to settle in Oman.

Pakistan
A medical examination is required of returning nationals, refugees and applicants for long-term stays.

Panama
An HIV test certificate is required of foreign nationals wishing to stay for more than 1 year, women wishing to work in "entertainment centres" and anyone wishing to extend an existing visa. HIV-positive people are refused entry.

Papua New Guinea
HIV testing required when applying for a work permit which is granted only if negative HIV test result can be presented.

Paraguay
Anyone applying for permanent residency in Paraguay is required to undergo HIV testing at the regional medical laboratory. No residence permit is granted if the test result is positive.

Peru
No specific entry restrictions. Those wishing to obtain a Peruvian marriage certificate are required to take an HIV test.

Philippines
No restrictions for short-term tourist stays lasting up to six months. Applicants for a permanent visa must undergo medical examination including an HIV test. This also applies to visitors who wish to extend an existing visa.

Poland
Applications for long-term stays require medical testing for HIV/AIDS.

Portugal
No restrictions.

Qatar
No HIV testing on entry. However, people whose HIV-status is known to the authorities

are refused entry. Applicants for a work or residence permit must present a negative HIV test certificate (the date of the certificate must not be older than six months).

Romania
No restrictions.

Russian Federation
HIV-positive people are not permitted to enter the Russian Federation. No HIV testing is required on entry for short-term tourist stays (up to three months).

Rwanda
There are no restriction entries to people living with HIV. However in the case of serious illness permission can be refused.

Solomon Islands
Entry can be denied if it becomes known, that the person in question has an infectious disease.

St Kitts and Nevis
Foreign nationals seeking permanent residence, undertaking study and those applying for work permits may be asked to undertake an HIV test.

Saudi Arabia
HIV testing on entry. HIV-positive foreign nationals are expelled.

Senegal
There are no restrictions regarding entry for HIV-positive persons.

Seychelles
The law states that foreigners are undesirable if they are carrying infections they are capable of infecting other people with. Applications for residency must be accompanied by medical certification proving that the applicant is in good health. Visitors who are working for the government must produce a negative HIV result. This does not apply to those working in the private sector or who are only applying for a short stay.

Singapore
No restrictions for short-term tourist stays lasting up to six months. Compulsory HIV testing when applying for work permits. The main group targeted is foreign domestic staff employed in Singapore. Foreign nationals with HIV-positive are expelled.

Slovakia
No restrictions for short-term tourist stays of up to three months.

South Africa
No restrictions for tourists with HIV. HIV testing required of all mine workers (irrespective of their positions).

Spain
Anyone seeking residence, or a work or student permit, must submit to a medical exam, which may include an HIV test.

Sri Lanka
No specific entry regulations for people with HIV. No questions asked about HIV on entry. However in cases in which an HIV infection is suspected, foreign nationals may be denied entry.

Sudan
Officially, people with HIV are not granted a visa and are not permitted to enter Sudan. A negative HIV test result must be presented at a Sudanese embassy or at Khartoum airport in order to obtain a visa. According to the embassy, this requirement is not enforced in practice.

Swaziland
There are no entry restrictions for people living with HIV.

Syria
Foreign nationals applying for work permits and foreign students must undergo an HIV test at one of three specified centres in Syria. A foreigner wishing to marry a Syrian national is required to take an HIV test.

Sweden
No restrictions for people with HIV. In case of doubt, the health authorities may oblige

a foreign national to undergo an HIV test. According to Swedish law, persons who come to Sweden and who have reason to believe they could be HIV-positive must consult a doctor and follow that doctor's advice.

Switzerland
No restrictions.

Tadjikistan
So far, it has been possible to enter the country without having to present an HIV test certificate. HIV testing is required for stays of more than 90 days.

Taiwan
An HIV test result must be presented by anyone wishing to stay longer than 90 days or applying for a residence or work permit. If the result is positive or if the person in question refuses to take the test, he/she is expelled.

Tanzania
No restrictions.

Thailand
According to the law, people with communicable diseases are not allowed to enter Thailand. However, no doctor's certificate is required at the border, so that an illness (as long as is not known) does not affect the granting of a visa. In some cases, a doctor's certificate including an HIV test has to be presented when applying for a visa extension (especially when applying for a long-term visa or a residence permit).

Trinidad and Tobago
All foreign nationals applying for residence or to stay more than one year must undergo a medical examination. Those found to be HIV-positive will be refused permission to stay.

Tunisia
There are no specific entry restrictions for HIV-positive people. Foreigners and students who intend to stay in the country for a long period are required to get tested on HIV.

Turkey
There are no entry or residence restrictions applicable to HIV-positive persons.

Turks and Caicos
All foreign nationals applying for work and residence permits must have a medical examination on arrival, including an HIV test.

Turkmenistan
No restrictions for short-term tourist stays. A positive test result may, however, lead to deportation.

Uganda
As a rule, health certificates or HIV test results do not have to be presented on entry or when applying for a long-term stay.

Ukraine
No restrictions.

United Arab Emirates
Foreign nationals aged 18 or above, applying for or renewing work or residence permits must undergo an HIV test. Entry will be refused to those who test positive.

United States of America
In principle, the USA refuses entry to foreign nationals known to be HIV positive. In exceptional cases, a stay of 30 days may be granted (for family visits, medical treatment, business travel or participation in a scientific, health-related conference).

HIV testing or a medical exam are not required. In the visa application form, the applicant has to say if he/she has a "communicable disease of public health significance". The visa will be denied if this is the case. An applicant who answers "no" despite better knowledge commits an immigration fraud, which leads to immigration prohibition.

HIV-positive foreign nationals lose their right to remain in the USA and are expelled if their status becomes known.

Uruguay
No restrictions for short-term tourist stays. If a routine examination reveals that a person is HIV positive, or if a person informs a doctor that he/she is HIV positive, that person must be reported to the Ministry of Health and undergo medical treatment. However this does not lead to expulsion or to any other immigration law restrictions.

Uzbekistan
Anyone staying for more than 15 days is required to provide an HIV certificate and longer term visitors must renew their HIV certificate after the first three months in the country, and annually thereafter.

Venezuela
No regulations regarding the entry or residence of people with HIV.

Vietnam
No specific entry or residence restrictions for people with HIV/AIDS. However the Vietnamese law requires HIV positive people to report to the health control authorities on entry.

Yemen (South)
No restrictions for tourist stays of up to two months. A negative test result has to be presented for stays of more than two months and HIV positive people are expelled immediately.

Zambia
No restrictions.

Zimbabwe
No restrictions.

Problems getting into the UK

Visitors `suspected of having AIDS' have been refused entry by individual immigration officers on questionable legal grounds.

The Home Office claims that the policy is only to exclude people if it is suspected that the person needs extensive medical treatment without being able to pay for it. For further information on UK immigration law and HIV see Immigration and asylum and HIV.

The best advice and help for anyone encountering difficulties is available from:

Joint Council for the Welfare of Immigrants
www.jcwi.org.uk - 020 7251 8708 - info@jcwi.org.uk

United Kingdom Immigration Advisory Service
http://www.iasuk.org - 020 7967 1200

Travelling with medication

If you are taking anti-HIV drugs you'll need to carry them with them when you travel. Customs officials often take a particular interest in medicines, and the discovery of anti-HIV drugs in the luggage of people with HIV has been the reason why many people have been refused entry to the USA and deported.

Some people get around the risk of travelling with their medication by taking the following action:

- They send their medication in advance. But make sure it arrives before you travel. Remember, post can be inspected by customs.

- Obtain medication in the country you want to travel to. However, this may not always be possible - or it could be extremely expensive.

If you carry your medication with you, have an answer ready about what the drugs are for. Some people say they are for cancer treatment. But remember, there's a reasonable chance that a customs official will have seen anti-HIV drugs before and won't be easily fooled. It might be helpful to have a letter from your doctor saying that the medicines you are carrying are for the treatment of a chronic medical condition and are for personal use. Make sure the letter doesn't mention HIV.

It might be very difficult, or even impossible, to get supplies of your medication once you've left home - even if you are just taking a short trip in the UK or Europe. So make sure you take enough of all your medicines with you to last the full duration of your trip. It might be wise to count out your medicines before you travel and to take a few additional doses just in case you get delayed.

Travelling across international time zones is likely to have implications for the time you take your medication. There are three options you may wish to consider. These include continuing to take your medicines at your UK time - but this could mean that you have to take your doses at inconvenient times. Another option is to gradually adjust the time you take your medicines, from UK time to the time in the country you are visiting. A third option might be altering your dose time to fit in with the time zone of the country you are visiting, but this could mean that there are some long intervals between doses as you adjust. It might be wise to talk over your plan with a doctor or pharmacist before you travel.

In good enough health to travel?

If you are planning a trip, then the chances are that your health will be up to it. But if you are feeling unwell, ask yourself honestly if you are in sufficiently good health to travel. Being ill away from home can be, at the very least, inconvenient, and it might be difficult to obtain specialist medical care or to come home early. What's more, if you are very ill, some airlines might refuse to carry you.

Travel insurance

General travel insurance policies generally exclude cover for pre-existing medical conditions, and some specifically exclude HIV. However it might be worth taking out cover just in case you have an illness that is unrelated to HIV, have an accident, lose your luggage or have something stolen.

What's more, some insurance companies are now willing to provide cover for people with HIV. Restrictions tend to apply, and premiums are often inflated.

NAM cannot recommend any particular provider of travel insurance company. It might be wise to shop around for a range of quotes and select the insurer which most meets your specific needs.

Freedom Travel Insurance
0870 774 3760
http://www.freedominsure.co.uk/

Easy Travel Insurance
0870 345 2222
www.hivtravelinsurance.com

Rothwell and Towler
01404 41234
www.travelfirst.co.uk

Reciprocal medical care

If you are travelling to another EU country you should obtain an European Health Insurance Card (EHIC) before you travel. This will provide you with free or reduced cost medical care in EU and some other countries. You can

apply for one online at
www.dh.gov.uk/policyandguidance/healthadvicefortravellers, or by calling
0845 606 2030 or from a Post Office. The form will tell you the exact
treatment which individual countries offer under the scheme. You may not get
free medical treatment in some countries.

Vaccinations

Find out if you need any special vaccinations and if it is safe for you to
receive them. Generally, people with HIV should not be given 'live' vaccines.
Talk to your doctor.

Treatment breaks and travel

Do not take a break from your HIV treatments or any other medicines you
have been prescribed without discussing it with your doctor in advance.

Further reading

- NAM factsheets, *Travelling with your HIV drugs* and
  Treatment interruption.

- 'Metal health and quality of life - travel' in NAM's *HIV
  andAIDS Reference Manual* (last updated in June
  2003).

- *Treatments and international travel,* booklet produced by
  the UK Coalition of People Living with HIV and AIDS.

Holiday hassles and HRT
by Caroline Guinness

A much-needed holiday. Tickets, passports, driving licence - all go in my hand luggage. I leave the toiletry bag out till the last minute. I don't care if everything else gets lost, but those pills must come with me on the plane. Into the bag they go.

The taxi's here right on time. Easy check-in at Gatwick, time to buy a few duty frees, which I've left space for in my hand luggage... I open it... stab of ice-cold fear... the toiletry bag... at home!

"Oh my God!" Husband goes pale. "Do you want to go back?" A few seconds' hesitation - "No! I'm getting on that plane."

A frantic call on the mobile (didn't forget that!) to the travel agent. No more flights till next week. FedEx will not courier medicines. A friend at home will try other courier companies.

I call my clinic. No, they do not know any doctors in Lanzarote but they will fax a letter and prescription to the travel rep there. I call the travel agent for their fax number. It turns out they are also the car hire company at Lanzarote Airport. My friend calls back, she has found a courier but the pills will have to go via Madrid and will not reach me till Monday (it is now Thursday). Our flight is being called.

Sitting on the plane, I realise that the travel rep and the car hire person will now know that I am HIV-positive. Oh great. In addition, I do not have my HRT - hormone hell for me and hubby, not a good prospect!

We land, find rep, she is fantastic. Married to a local doctor, she has spent the last two hours trying to sort things out - no go. The clinic system is like the UK - they don't just hand over HIV pills willy-nilly. She takes me to the airport pharmacy. A sweet man hands over my HRT, which is a major relief, but no HIV combo.

Weather perfect, accommodation divine. I call my clinic, they tell me not to panic, things should be OK. I have been adherent for four years, undetectable and feeling well. There might be a small 'blip'. Just make sure to take my pills as soon as they arrive, make sure I have bloods done as soon as I return. I have done everything I can.

I do not feel stressed. In fact, I feel fantastic. Have my first good night's sleep in years. Have my first 'real' dreams. Wake up refreshed for the first time in years. Husband says he can see my shoulders dropping. I feel light and NORMAL.

Monday, I call Madrid. My pills have left there and are on their way to Las Palmas, then another flight to Lanzarote, and should be there by 4.15pm. I do not feel relieved. Strangely sad, in fact.

"Why?" my husband asks.

"Well, let me try and explain. Imagine you lost a leg and were given an artificial one. You are grateful for the mobility it gives you. Then for four days your leg grows back, but only for four days. Does that make it clearer?"

Pills in my hand, swallow. Within two hours I am feeling weird, slight hallucinations, sick. That night 'the dreams'. Wake feeling vile. How come? The sun is still shining, I'm still on holiday. Yet that low level of anxiety is back. Now I know it's not me, it's the efavirenz.

I know what it is to have AIDS; I know these things are a better alternative. I should be grateful, but still I grieve. I realise, now, why we are entitled to Disability Living Allowance. You may not see the disability, but this is what it feels like. It's real.

A week later, I am back at my Clinic. "How do you feel?" They ask anxiously. "Fine," I reply. "You look great." I always do with a suntan!

I see my consultant on 20th March. No viral 'blip', thank God, but psychologically, it has not just been a 'blip', it's been an explosion. I must discuss (again) a Structured Treatment Interruption. Oh for a cure!

This first appeared in issue 78 of Positive Nation, May 2002. Many thanks to both Caroline and Positive Nation for giving permission to reprint it.

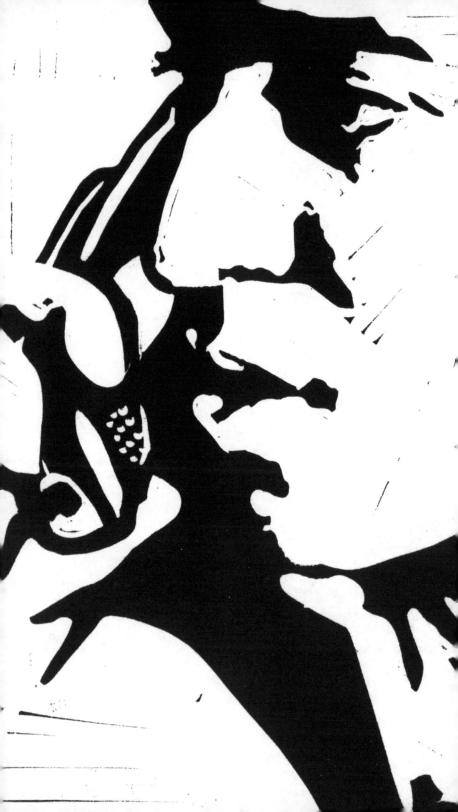

Work

In this chapter you'll find information on

Returning to work, training or study.

Your employment rights if you have HIV.

The 1996 edition of *Living with HIV and AIDS* contained hardly any information on working if you are HIV-positive. Until effective anti-HIV treatment became available, HIV services were largely geared towards helping people claim their state benefits and managing retirement from work on the basis of ill health.

It's an indication of just how successful anti-HIV treatment can be that many people with HIV are now either remaining in the workplace or thinking about returning to work or study.

Work can have many advantages, including stimulation, enjoyment, a sense of accomplishment, company and friendship - and a regular financial income.

There can, however, be some very real difficulties returning to work after having a prolonged period of time off due to illness. There's also a chance that you might encounter some difficulties in the workplace related to your HIV infection.

Going back to work

An early, and important decision you'll need to make is what work do you wish to do?

You might want to pick up where you left off. However, particularly if it's a long time since you were last employed, starting again where you left off might not be an option.

Alternatively, you might want to use your return to work as an opportunity to change direction and enter a new line of work.

For some people with HIV, it's not a question of 'returning' to work, but of entering the workplace for the first time.

Whatever situation you're in, there's a good chance you'll need some training to help you prepare, both practically and mentally, for work.

Training

If you want to gain new skills or experience, you could perhaps do some voluntary work, enrol in a course, or register on a training scheme.

Volunteering can provide an opportunity to gain new skills and at the same time gain a familiarity with working conditions. The routine of volunteering can also help simulate the routine of working, and if you are volunteering in an area similar to the one in which you'd like to work, it can provide an opportunity to discover if this really is something you'd like to do.

Many people find that volunteering helps boost their self-confidence and acts as a useful bridge back to work.

Studying

To gain employment in your area of interest, it might be necessary to gain specific skills or a qualification. Colleges and universities around the country have part-time study opportunities for adults, ranging from open access courses with no entry requirements to higher degrees.

As well as equipping you with skills and qualifications, studying can help focus your attention on what job or career you'd like to undertake, and build your confidence.

Help for applying for jobs

Local job centres and some HIV organisations can help you develop or enhance your job application and interview skills.

The impact of returning to work or study

If you left work a number of years ago, or have never worked, the prospect of getting a job can be daunting. Your confidence might be low, you might feel left behind or deskilled. Although you may be able to go straight into full-time employment, a more realistic plan might be to undertake some part-time work, either paid or voluntary, or study, and find a working balance that suits you.

The impact that working or studying can have on your benefits can be a real worry. Many people with HIV have reported being in a 'benefits trap'. If you qualify for the maximum rate of benefits, you might actually be financially worse off if you return to work, unless the job is very well paid.

You might also be deterred from thinking about work or study because you are uncertain about how long you'll remain healthy, or are worried that working might damage your health.

Working with HIV

Disclosure

Unless you're working in certain healthcare professions, there's absolutely no requirement for you to tell your employer that you're HIV-positive.

Nevertheless, you may choose to tell your employer in the hope that this will lead to a more supportive working environment. However, you may prefer to keep information about your health confidential in order to avoid discrimination or having to deal with colleagues' attitudes towards HIV.

If you need time off because of illness or for hospital appointments think about how you are going to explain this without disclosing your HIV status.

HIV testing

There's no law to stop an employer asking for an HIV test as part of a company medical for new employees. However, they've no right to see the result of the test result without your consent.

The only way an employer can ask an existing employee to take an HIV test is if the initial terms and conditions of a job said that this would be the case.

Employment rights

The Disability Discrimination Act provides important workplace protection to people with HIV from the moment of their HIV diagnosis. These rights are on top of those provided by other legislation.

Basically, it is unlawful for an employer with 15 or more employees to:

- Discriminate against an HIV-positive person in recruitment and selection unless this can be 'justified'.

- Give an HIV-positive person less favourable treatment (including access to promotion, training and transfers, as well as dismissal and selection for redundancy) unless this can be 'justified'.

- Fail to make 'reasonable' adjustments to the work environment to enable an HIV-positive person to work.

Can my employer sack me because I'm ill due to HIV?

UK Government guidelines in the booklet *AIDS and the Workplace* state that:

> "HIV infection alone does not affect people's ability to do their job until they develop illnesses that make them unfit... If they later become ill, they should be treated like anyone else with a life-threatening illness. Only if their illness affects their ability to do the job should their employer seek medical advice."

The only way this advice will have changed since the Disability Discrimination Act is that the employer must have considered reasonable adjustments before dismissing you as a result of HIV-related illness.

If you are dismissed because you are unable to do the job, the employer must have sufficient evidence upon which to base that decision. This involves, preferably, both a report from the employee's doctor and an examination by a doctor on behalf of the employer.

If you are physically unable to carry out your contractual job, then the employer should consider the possibility of a move to different duties. The likelihood of there being suitable alternative employment will depend largely on the size of the firm involved. Furthermore, there is no duty for the employer to create alternative employment.

Seek legal advice if your employer is causing you difficulties in relation to time off for sickness.

Further reading

- A good place to start is the UK Coalition of People Living With HIV and AIDS's "Into work guide" which can be accessed on their website www.ukcoalition.org. A printed copy of the guide can be obtained by calling 020 7564 2180.

- 'Employment and HIV' in NAM's *HIV and AIDS Reference Manual*.

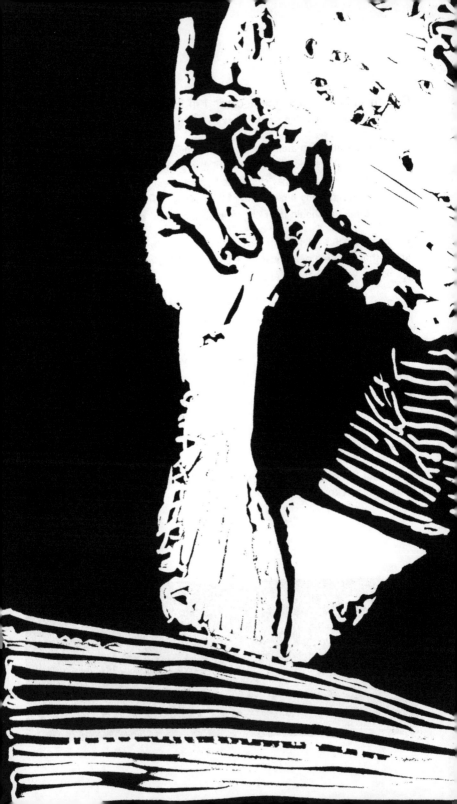

HIV and the law

by James Chalmers

This chapter provides information on

The law and the confidentiality of
medical records.

HIV transmission and the criminal law.

Immigration and asylum law.

The Disability Discrimination Act.

Introduction

This section was written in early 2006. It was accurate at the time of writing, but the law relating to HIV is subject to change, both because of court rulings and legislation. It's important to obtain specialist legal advice from a lawyer.

Confidentiality

Introduction

Confidential information may be protected by law. The House of Lords, the highest court in the land, confirmed in 2004 that "a duty of confidence will arise whenever the party subject to the duty is in a situation where he knows or ought to know that the other person can reasonably expect his privacy to be respected."

But a ruling from 1990 set out limitations to this principle:

- It only applies to information which is actually confidential. Once information enters the public domain, it is no longer protected by confidentiality.

- It does not apply to useless or trivial information.

- Although it is in the public interest that confidential information should be protected, that public interest may sometimes be outweighed by another public interest favouring disclosure. In such cases, the public interest in confidentiality must be balanced against the public interest in disclosure.

The last one of these exceptions is probably the most important in the context of HIV.

Confidentiality and HIV

As early as 1988 a case involving two doctors showed that HIV was covered by confidentiality. An unknown health authority employee (or employees) passed information regarding these doctors' HIV status to a newspaper reporter. The newspaper intended to publish an article identifying the doctors concerned and describing their condition. The health authority sought a court order preventing the newspaper from publishing the information, or using it in any other way, which was granted.

The court noted that there was a public interest in the freedom of the press, and also accepted that there was some public interest in the information which the newspaper sought to publish. However, "those public interests [were] substantially outweighed when measured against the public interests in relation to loyalty and confidentiality both generally and with particular reference to AIDS patients' hospital records."

Confidentiality and HIV/AIDS

As early as 1988 a case involving two doctors showed that HIV was covered by confidentiality. An unknown health authority employee (or employees) passed that information regarding the doctors' HIV status to a newspaper reporter. The newspaper intended to publish an article identifying the doctors concerned and describing their condition. The health authority sought a court order preventing the newspaper from publishing the information, or using it in any other way, which was granted.

The court noted that there was a public interest in the freedom of the press, and also accepted that there was some public interest in the information which the newspaper sought to publish. However, "those public interests [were] substantially outweighed when measured against the public interests in relation to loyalty and confidentiality both generally and with particular reference to AIDS patients' hospital records."

Disclosure of confidential medical information in the public interest

Confidential medical information may sometimes be disclosed in the public interest. For example, in 1990 a court considered the case of a patient detained in a mental hospital, whose psychiatrist had sent a report on his condition to the Secretary of State suggesting that he should not be released. The court decided that the public interest in protecting the safety of others outweighed the public interest in preserving an individual's right to confidentiality.

In certain circumstances, this principle may be relied upon to justify the disclosure of information about a person's HIV-positive status without their consent. The General Medical Council's Guidance to Doctors on Serious Communicable Diseases (1997) states as follows (paras 26-27):

"You may disclose information about a patient, whether living or dead, in order to protect a person from risk of death or serious harm. For example, you may disclose information to a known sexual contact of a patient with HIV where you have reason to think that the patient has not informed that person, and cannot be persuaded to do so. In such circumstances you should tell the patient before you make the disclosure, and you must be prepared to justify a decision to disclose information. You must not disclose information to others, for example relatives, who have not been, and are not, at risk of infection."

The guidance also notes that confidential medical information may be disclosed to other health care workers if failure to disclose would put them at a serious risk of death or serious harm (para 19).

There are specific provisions about the confidentiality which attaches to a diagnosis of infection with a sexually transmitted infection: the National Health Service (Venereal Diseases) Regulations 1974. There is some doubt about the exact meaning and effect of these regulations, and as this book went to press, the Department of Health was undertaking a consultation exercise on their future.

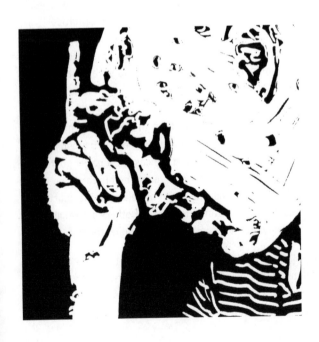

HIV transmission and the criminal law

Introduction

Up until relatively recently, it was thought that the transmission of HIV (at least through consensual sexual intercourse, or the sharing of drug-injecting equipment) could not amount to a criminal offence in the UK. In England and Wales, this was because the relevant offence - "unlawfully and maliciously inflicting grievous bodily harm" - had been interpreted by the courts in the nineteenth century as being restricted to cases where one person had attacked another, for example by striking a blow or using a knife. However, that interpretation of the offence changed over time, and it was gradually recognised that the offence could apply to any case of "causing" harm.

The first successful prosecution for HIV transmission in England and Wales was brought against Mohammed Dica, who was convicted of two counts of unlawfully and maliciously inflicting grievous bodily harm in October 2003. Although his conviction was later quashed by the Court of Appeal (because the judge had misdirected the jury on the question of consent), the court accepted that the transmission of HIV could, in certain circumstances, amount to a criminal offence, and Dica was convicted of a single count at a retrial. A similar conclusion had already been reached in Scotland in 2001 (where a different system of criminal law applies), when Stephen Kelly was convicted of having 'recklessly injured' his former partner by infecting her with HIV.

It should be stressed at the outset that prosecutions for the transmission of HIV are likely to be unusual. There have been two in Scotland since Stephen Kelly's conviction in 2001 (neither of which went to trial), while there have been five convictions in England following the Dica case. The Crown Prosecution Service was, at the time of writing, about to start a consultation exercise on the circumstances in which prosecutions might be appropriate.

The offence is not, it should be noted, limited to HIV, but might extend to any other sexually transmitted infection which could be considered to amount to "grievous bodily harm".

The "state of mind" required for the offence

There is no question of any person being liable of a criminal offence simply because they have transmitted HIV to another person. To be guilty of any serious criminal offence, a person must have acted with a culpable state of mind - which lawyers refer to as *mens rea*. The *mens rea* required for the offence of inflicting grievous bodily harm is intention or recklessness. In other words, for a conviction, it would be necessary to show that the defendant intended to infect the other party with HIV, or that they were reckless as to this possibility - that is, that the defendant was aware of the risk of infection. This would also be necessary in Scotland for the offence of "reckless injury" of which Stephen Kelly was convicted.

It is theoretically possible, therefore, that a person could be guilty of this offence even if they had not received a positive result from an HIV test. It would, however, be necessary to show that they were aware of a significant risk that they might be HIV-positive - for example, if they had previously been regularly engaged in unprotected intercourse with a person or persons whom they knew to be HIV-positive. While a prosecution in such a case would be unlikely, it should be made clear that avoiding taking an HIV test does not provide immunity from criminal prosecution. One of the English prosecutions to date involved a man who had never taken an HIV test, but had been diagnosed with other sexually transmitted infections, warned that he was at very high risk of being HIV-positive and had failed thereafter to attend an appointment for testing.

What is the effect of consent?
In quashing Mohammed Dica's convictions after his first trial, the Court of Appeal ruled that, where a person chooses to consent to the risk of HIV transmission (that is, they know that their sexual partner is HIV-positive and choose to have unprotected intercourse regardless of this fact), then that will be a valid defence to a criminal prosecution. This would not, however, apply in the unlikely event that the consenting party had actually *wanted* to become infected with HIV (and the other party had intended this to happen). It is thought that the Scottish courts would take the same view.

What if condoms are used, or high-risk activities avoided?
What is the situation if a person who is HIV-positive does not disclose this fact to their sexual partner, but uses condoms, and HIV is nevertheless transmitted? In the Dica case, the Court of Appeal suggested that the use of condoms might mean that the HIV-positive person could not be said to have acted "recklessly", and so therefore would not have the state of mind required for the offence. Similarly, if the parties refrain from high-risk sexual

activities, again, "recklessness" would not be present. A problem does arise, however, in relation to unprotected oral sex, which is not normally considered high-risk but does present a more than negligible risk. It is thought that it would not be caught by the criminal law, but the exact position is unclear.

What if transmission does not occur?

In England and Wales, if an HIV-positive person has unprotected sexual intercourse without disclosing their serostatus, but the other party does not become infected, then a prosecution would be very unlikely. It is possible that there could be a prosecution for an attempt to inflict grievous bodily harm in such a case, but the prosecutor would have to show that the defendant actually intended to transmit the disease. It would not be enough to show that the positive person was simply reckless as to the possibility of the disease being transmitted. In Scotland, however, it is at least theoretically possible that there could be a prosecution for "reckless endangerment" in the absence of actual transmission.

A duty to disclose?

Because consent is a valid defence, it seems fair to say that the Dica case effectively places a legal duty on HIV-positive persons to disclose their HIV-status before engaging in high-risk sexual activities.

Immigration and asylum law

UK immigration law is governed by the Immigration Act 1971. This has since been amended by subsequent pieces of legislation, particularly the Nationality, Immigration and Asylum Act 2002. More specific regulations are contained in the Immigration Rules, which are made by the Home Secretary and laid before Parliament. These are available online at www.ind.homeoffice.gov.uk.

This section provides a brief overview of immigration and asylum law as it affects people with HIV. It is, however, in no way a comprehensive statement of the law and is no substitute for specialist advice. Immigration law is complex, changes frequently and it can be important to meet deadlines and follow correct procedures in order to preserve your legal rights. For that reason, anyone facing a problem concerned with this area of the law should seek proper advice at the earliest possible opportunity.

The relevance of being HIV-positive

Neither the legislation nor the Immigration Rules specifically mention HIV. The UK has not adopted a ban on persons with HIV entering the United Kingdom, unlike a small number of other countries (including, most significantly, the USA). HIV-positive status may nevertheless be relevant to asylum and immigration decisions, depending on the type of decision concerned and the situation of the individual concerned. It is essential here to distinguish between different categories of persons. There are, essentially, two questions: first, can being HIV-positive or having been diagnosed with AIDS be a barrier to entering the UK? And secondly, where a person is already in the UK, can being HIV-positive or diagnosed with AIDS be a reason which justifies continuing to remain in the UK when that individual would otherwise be required to leave?

People not subject to UK immigration law

Most obviously, British citizens are not subject to immigration law. Nor are citizens of other states within the European Economic Area (EEA), who have specific rights of entry to the UK. Certain Commonwealth citizens also have a "right of abode" in the UK. For these persons, being HIV-positive should not affect entry into the UK.

Any other person, however, requires leave to enter the UK (Immigration Rules, para 7).

Leave to enter the UK and HIV-positive status

Where a person requires leave to enter, the UK's current (and long-standing) policy is that the fact that a person is HIV-positive, or has AIDS, is not in itself a ground for refusing leave to enter the UK. (Leave may, of course, still be refused if that person does not otherwise qualify for leave under the Rules.) However, the effect which a medical condition may have on a person's ability to support himself or herself is a factor which the Immigration Officer may take into account in deciding whether to grant leave to enter.

A person who intends to remain in the UK for more than six months should normally be referred to the Medical Inspector for examination (Immigration Rules, para 36), and the inspector will be expected to estimate the cost of any treatment which may be required so that this can be considered by the Immigration Officer.

Entering the UK for medical treatment

A person may seek leave to enter or remain in the UK in order to receive private medical treatment. The relevant criteria are set out at paras 51-56 of the Immigration Rules. In particular, it will be necessary for such a person to show that he or she has sufficient funds to meet the costs of treatment. It is also necessary that the applicant "can show, if required to do so, that any proposed course of treatment is of finite duration" (para 51(iii)). It would not, therefore, normally be possible to use these provisions to seek entry to the UK for ongoing HIV or AIDS treatment, although they could, for example, apply for leave to enter to seek treatment for an HIV-related illness. Leave to enter for private medical treatment will, in practice, only be a realistic option for the relatively wealthy. NHS treatment is not automatically free for those from overseas.

Can HIV be a ground for remaining in the UK?

Where a person is entitled to apply for leave to remain on grounds unrelated to their HIV-positive status, then the same principle as noted earlier applies: the fact that someone is HIV-positive or has AIDS is not in itself a basis for refusing that application.

However, there may be cases where a person has no other grounds to remain in the UK, but wishes to seek discretionary leave to remain on the basis that they will not receive adequate medical treatment in their home country.

Such applications may be bolstered by reference to the European Convention on Human Rights, article 3 of which provides that "no one shall be subjected to torture or to inhuman or degrading treatment or punishment". In the case of D v United Kingdom (1997) 24 EHRR 423, the European Court of Human Rights held that it would be a breach of article 3 for the UK government to deport a prisoner, very close to death as the result of AIDS, to his home country of St Kitts where care would be inadequate and he would be at a real risk of dying under most distressing circumstances.

However, in 2005, the House of Lords confirmed that the decision in D will be applied only in very exceptional circumstances. In N v Secretary of State for the Home Department [2005] UKHL 31, N, a Ugandan citizen entered the UK claiming asylum. She was diagnosed as being HIV-positive while in the UK. Her claim for asylum was unsuccessful, and she claimed that to return her to Uganda would violate her rights under article 3 of the

European Convention. The court rejected this argument, holding that article 3 would not be violated solely on the basis that the medical facilities in the country to which a person was to be sent did not match those in the country which that person was to be removed from.

Following the decision in N, current Home Office guidelines state that "where the claimant would be in no worse position than the majority of people in his country of origin who suffer from the same condition, then a grant of Discretionary Leave would not normally be appropriate as it would not be an exceptional case." (Immigration Directorate Instructions, chapter 1, section 8, part 3.4.) It is important, therefore, that if an application for discretionary leave is to be made, that care is taken to prepare a full and detailed case explaining the relevant circumstances.

Asylum law

In an appropriate case, it is possible that an HIV-positive person who has a "well-founded fear of persecution" because of their HIV status if they are returned to their home country might be able to claim asylum on that basis. Again, it would be essential to prepare a full and detailed case in support of such an application.

Disability Discrimination Act (DDA)

The Disability Discrimination Act 1995 provided some limited protection against discrimination faced by persons with HIV and AIDS, but this was limited in scope because the Act did not automatically apply to a person who was HIV-positive. This was changed by the Disability Discrimination Act 2005, which updated and amended the 1995 Act. As a result of the 2005 Act, a person with HIV is "deemed" to be a disabled person for the purposes of the legislation.

The Act protects disabled persons against discrimination in a variety of fields, including employment, the provision of goods, facilities and services, the disposal of premises (which includes granting leases or sub-leases), education and public transport.

In respect of employment, an employer will be said to discriminate against an employee if "for a reason which relates to the disabled person's disability, he treats him less favourably than he treats or would treat others" and "he cannot show that the treatment in question is justified". In most cases, it is unlikely that an employer would be able to show that less favourable treatment could be justified on the basis of HIV infection alone. For example, in a case in 2005, an HIV-positive carer - who worked with men with aggressive behavioural difficulties - was dismissed by his employers, who argued that there was a risk that he could be bitten by clients who could then be infected with HIV. He took action under the Disability Discrimination Act, arguing (amongst other things) that this risk was negligible, given that cases of HIV being transmitted by biting are exceptionally rare. A tribunal ruled in his favour.

In respect of the provision of services (including the provision of goods or facilities), it is unlawful for a service provider not to provide to a disabled person services which he provides to members of the public, or to discriminate in the standard of service or the terms on which the service is provided. Again, proving discrimination requires that the service provider cannot show that the less favourable treatment is justified.

The Act also places persons such as employers and service providers under duties to make reasonable adjustments to avoid disadvantaging persons with disabilities. Where these duties are not complied with, the failure to do so is not a basis for arguing that the less favourable treatment of the disabled person was justified.

Further reading

- James Chalmers, 'Criminalising HIV infection,' *AIDS Treatment Update* 131.
- Edwin Bernard, 'Criminalising HIV transmission: update,' *AIDS Treatment Update* 148.
- 'The law and HIV' in NAM's *HIV and AIDS Reference Manual*.

Anger

I wasn't really surprised when I found out I had HIV, after all I went to have an HIV test because I had all the symptoms you get soon after you're infected with HIV - a sore throat, headache, fever, and patchy red rash. The doctor who I saw before I had the bloods taken for my test didn't seem to think there was going to be much doubt about the outcome and told me to prepare for a positive result. Nevertheless, I was still a bit numbed by the result.

This numbness gradually mutated into anger. It was quite unlike any anger I'd ever felt before and quite literally consumed me. There were two focuses for this anger. First of all, there was myself. My diagnosis with HIV provided an opportunity to beat myself up, something which the homophobia I experienced throughout my adolescence and early adulthood had made me expert at.

But most of all I was furious with the man who gave me HIV. Up until I met him, I'd taken excellent care of my sexual health; I'd never even had the most minor of sexually transmitted infections. We used condoms the first few times we had sex, but he made it very clear that he didn't like them. I know that people reading this will say, "well, you should have insisted." But before you pass judgment, ask yourself: have you ever been influenced into doing something you've subsequently regretted against your better judgment?

Another issue was that he was bigger than me - not physically, but emotionally. I was 24 and he was 30. I know it doesn't sound like a big difference, but in terms of life experience and confidence it really was.

Well, we had unprotected sex - not once, but many times. I even initiated some of it. The sex felt good and I believed it was strengthening our physical and emotional intimacy. Within a year, I developed what turned out to be an HIV seroconversion illness. The relationship had broken down by then, and when I contacted him to tell him I had HIV he couldn't have been less concerned.

I tried to take full responsibility for my infection with HIV; after all I'd seen all the safer sex ads. But I still couldn't stop feeling so angry with him, particularly when I subsequently found out that he was believed to have given HIV to an earlier boyfriend.

My feelings of betrayal and anger were intensified by a kind of righteousness - I wanted this man stopped before he could give HIV to somebody else and ruin their life. The intensity of my anger was overpowering, indeed for about a year after finding out I had HIV it was this anger rather than anything HIV did to my body that affected my health and quality of life.

A fit of drunken rage in front of some friends prompted me to admit that I was being damaged by my anger and I sought some professional support. Initially I wanted to talk through my options about getting even and obtaining some justice. To put it simply, I wanted the man who gave me HIV punished; I told myself it would help redress the balance, I was sick and tired of punishing myself. Retribution in some form, I assured myself, would draw a line under my diagnosis and allow me to move on.

In the first few counselling sessions all I could talk about was the deep knot of fury that was tightening within me. But, as the therapy progressed, I realised that I was feeding and intensifying this anger and that doing this was exhausting and damaging me. Focusing all my energy and emotions on a quest for justice meant that I wasn't dealing at all with my HIV diagnosis and was using my desire for justice and revenge as a way of separating myself off from other people with HIV - I almost felt as if I had 'good HIV'. What's more, I just wasn't looking after my physical or emotional health, and more or less absolved myself of responsibility for my own wellbeing - I just felt that what had happened to me wasn't my fault and could be excused more or less any responsibility for looking after myself.

Well, I gradually worked out that I wasn't that different from other people with HIV - we all had an infection, that didn't discriminate in terms of moral worthiness. In addition, I realised that even if my desire to see my ex-partner punished was accomplished, I'd still be infected with HIV, and I needed to get to terms with what this really meant and start living with the virus and all its ramifications on a day-to-day basis.

Over the coming months I also began to gradually admit that it had taken two of us to have unprotected sex. There'd been safer sex information around for as long as I'd been sexually aware. I knew how to avoid HIV; I knew that I had responsibility for my own health; I knew not to assume anything about my partners' HIV status. The counselling helped me to start understand how my own abilities to look after myself had been eroded by the chronic homophobia I experienced throughout my adolescence. To be honest, I was so emotionally ill-equipped that, even if I hadn't contracted HIV when I did, I'd have been infected with it later on.

I'm writing this years after my diagnosis. At the time I was told that it was unlikely the law could do anything to punish the person I held responsible for my HIV infection. If it had been an option, would I have complained to the police? Well, he was a pretty unpleasant guy, but focusing on a desire for revenge did me no good what so ever. I've subsequently got on with my life; sure I've still got issues about having HIV (one of which is that I now feel semi-criminalised by being sexually active and HIV-positive), but I know for certain that these wouldn't have been solved by seeing the person who infected me imprisoned.

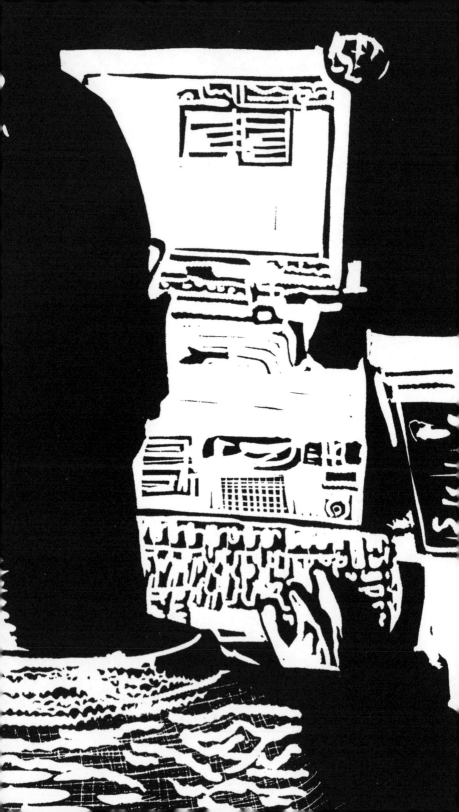

Finding information

In this chapter you'll find information on

National helplines you may find useful.

Some key national organisations that
represent the interests of people with HIV.

A selection of HIV-related websites.

There are many organisations around the UK offering services and information to people with HIV.

NAM publishes the *UK AIDS Directory* every year. It includes information on HIV clinics and services providers throughout the UK. You can also search for HIV clinics on NAM's website www.aidsmap.com.

There have been a lot of changes in the HIV voluntary sector, with many organisations either merging with other HIV charities or closing altogether.

To find out what HIV services are available near you, a good place to start would be to call one of the national helplines listed below or talk to one of the professionals you are currently receiving HIV services from.

The quality of HIV information on the internet ranges from excellent to mad, bad, and dangerous to know. Details of a few key sites are listed below.

National Helplines

National Drugs Helpline
0800 776 600 (freephone)
Every day 24 hours

National free helpline offering advice, information and referrals on all drug issues including HIV and AIDS.

National Sexual Health Helpline
0800 567 123 (freephone)
Every day 24 hours

National telephone helpline answering calls on all aspects of sexual health including HIV.

NHS Direct
0845 4647 (calls charged at local rate)
Every day 24 hours
www.nhsdirect.nhs.uk

NHS Direct provides a 24-hour nurse advice and health information service, providing confidential information on what to do if you are feeling ill, general information on health conditions, local health services such as GPs and late night chemists, and support and self help groups.

THT Direct

0845 1221 200 (calls charged at local rate)
Mon - Fri, 10am - 10pm
Sat - Sun, 12noon - 6pm
www.tht.org.uk

A gateway to HIV information, services and support provided by the Terrence Higgins Trust (THT), the largest HIV charity in the UK. THT provide extensive published information and a wide range of support and advocacy services.

THT currently offers services in London, Bath, Birmingham, Brighton, Bristol, Cardiff, Coventry, Eastbourne, Essex, Leeds, Oxford, Surrey, Swansea, Swindon and Wolverhampton. Details of the services available at each centre and how to access them can be obtained from THT direct.

i-Base Treatment Information Phoneline

0808 800 6013 (freephone)
Mon - Weds, 12noon - 4pm
www.i-base.org

Phoneline providing confidential information on HIV treatment.

Hepatitis C information line

0800 451451
Open from 10am-10pm, seven days a week.

Key self-help, advocacy and specialist groups

African HIV Policy Network (AHPN)

New City Cloisters, 196 Old Street, London EC1V PFR
020 7017 8910
info@ahpn.org
www.ahpn.org

The African HIV Policy Network (AHPN) is an umbrella organisation which represents African community groups addressing HIV/AIDS and sexual health throughout the UK.

GMFA

Unit 43 Eurolink Centre, 49 Effra Road, London SW2 1BZ
020 7738 6872
gmfa@gmfa.org.uk
www.metromate.org.uk

GMFA (Gay Men Fighting AIDS) is a London-based, volunteer-led gay men's health organisation. Volunteers are supported and trained to develop and execute health interventions for gay men. GMFA's HIV prevention interventions include workshops, press adverts, a newsletter and this website. Their interventions to improve the health of HIV positive gay men include press work and workshops. GMFA's general health work includes smoking cessation workshops.

The Haemophilia Society

First Floor, Petersham House, 57a Hatton Garden, London, EC1N 8JG
020 7831 1020
0800 018 6068 (freephone helpline)
Mon-Fri, 10am - 4pm
info@haemophilia.org.uk
www.haemophilia.org.uk

The Society is involved in providing advocacy, information, support and advice to all those living with haemophilia and other blood clotting disorders. The Society also supports those with blood clotting disorders and viral hepatitis as a result of their NHS treatment with infected blood products.

NAZ Project

Palingswick House (annex), 241 King St, London W6 9LP
020 8741 1879
npl@naz.org.uk
www.naz.org.uk

Naz Project London provides sexual health and HIV prevention and support services to South Asian, Middle Eastern, North African, Horn of African and Latin American Communities.

Naz aims to educate and empower communities to face up to the challenges of sexual health and the AIDS pandemic, and to mobilise the support networks that exist for people living with HIV/AIDS.

Positively Women
347-349 City Road, London EC1V 1LR
020 7713 0444
020 7713 0222
Helpline Monday - Friday, 10am - 1pm and 2pm - 4pm
info@positivelywomen.org.uk
www.positivelywomen.org.uk

A national charity working to life of women and families affected by HIV.

UK Coalition of People Living with HIV and AIDS (UKC)
250 Kennington Lane, London SE11 5RD
020 7564 2180
reception@ukcoalition.org
www.ukcoalition.org

UKC is a group of people living with HIV and AIDS, campaigning, researching and providing services by and for people with HIV. Publishers of *Positive Nation* the UK's HIV and sexual health magazine.

Websites

AEGIS
www.aegis.com

The most extensive collection of links on AIDS, with searchable electronic versions of many newsletters and a vast catalogue of news stories, plus discussion forums.

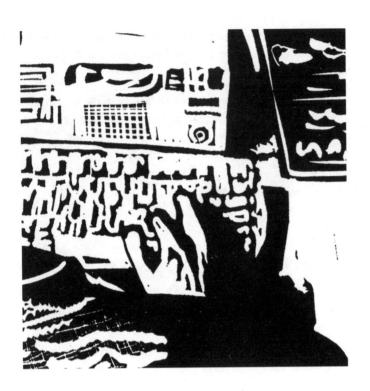

AIDS
www.aidsonline.com

An influential medical journal sponsored by the International AIDS Society, with free access to abstracts, which provide a summary of the key findings of research. Full text access only available to subscribers.

aidsmap.com
www.aidsmap.com

NAM's website. On this site you can find more original, daily news on developments in the world of HIV than any other HIV website. The site also includes completely searchable databases of HIV treatment and care, worldwide HIV organisation listings, and one of the most comprehensive ranges of patient information available on the web.

American Foundation for AIDS Research (AMFAR)
www.amfar.org

A good searchable treatment database, excellent news and analysis and a nice simple design.

AVERT
www.avert.org

AVERT is an international HIV and AIDS charity based in the UK, with the aim of AVERTing HIV and AIDS worldwide.

Clinical Care Options for HIV
www.clinicaloptions.com/hiv

A site targeted at HIV medical professionals.

HIVandHepatitis.com
www.hivandhepatitis.com

This site concentrates on news and conference reports, largely targeted at medical professionals.

HIVInsite
www.hivinsite.com

The electronic version of the AIDS Knowledge Base, a textbook developed by physicians at San Francisco General Hospital. The site also contains databases on trials, drug interactions and side effects, as well as news stories and a library of reports on prevention issues.

International AIDS Society
www.ias.se

Website of the International AIDS Society which includes daily news. The site also makes available abstracts of conferences organised by the International AIDS Society including the International AIDS Conference.

Medscape
www.medscape.com/hiv-aidshome

Another site designed to provide doctors with continuing medical education on HIV. The site also provides daily news and conference coverage.

The Body
www.thebody.com

An extensive collection of articles from HIV newsletters and other publications around the world, and an exclusive "Ask the Experts" forum for you to put questions to the leading doctors.

UNAIDS
www.unaids.com

United Nations AIDS Programme - information about the activities of the programme, access to policy documents and records of UNAIDS-sponsored interventions; statistics on the global epidemic.

T-cell chronicles
http://www.tcellchronicles.org

Creating awareness and empowering the global HIV and AIDS community through the written word.

DIPEx
www.dipex.org/hiv

The DIPEx HIV module is a unique public access website containing video clips of interviews in which 50 people describe their experience of HIV. The website includes gay men and black Africans (the two groups most affected by HIV in Britain) talking about their experience of living with the infection. The website will be organised with 25 'chapters' on how people cope (e.g. mental health, gaining strength, sex, getting health care, getting support) and will contain moving firsthand accounts. It is being built 'from the ground up' using established methods of qualitative research and will be launched in late 2006.

Index

#

3TC (lamivudine, *Epivir*) 91, 189
   as a cause of neuropathy 142
   as a cause of nausea 133
   treatment for hepatitis B 94, 168

A

abacavir (*Ziagen*) 91, 296
   as a cause of nausea 133
   hypersensitivity reaction 130
   switching to because of fat loss . . . . .
   . . . . .103, 137
   use of to prevent dementia 274
abdomen .159
aciclovir .159
acupuncture 201, 235
adefovir (*Hespera*)
   treatment for hepatitis B 168
adherence 118, 101
   and cocaine use 227
   and ecstasy use 230
   and ketamine use 231
   and life-style 122
   and LSD use 231
   and mental health 120
   and methamphetamine use 228
   and money worries 121
   and pill burden 120
   and side-effects 120
   and your life-style 120
   diary 124

   impact of going on holiday, travelling .
  124
   importance of 118
   jogging memory 124
   level to aim for 119
   missed and late doses, experiences of .
  7
   missed doses 97
   personal experiences of 126, 205
   pill boxes 124
   practicising 124
   strategies to improve 124
   support from your HIV clinic . . . .
   . . . . .59, 123
advocacy .59
aegis.com 371
aerobic exercise 267
African HIV Policy
Network (AHPN) 369
AIDS .32, 34
   annual number of deaths
   in the UK 166, 242
   annual number of
   diagnoses in the UK 166, 242
   good health after being
   diagnosed with 35
   medical journal of 372
   tuberculosis is an
   AIDS-defining illness 165
AIDS deaths
   fall in since introduction
   of HAART 36
AIDS Treatment Update 94
aidsmap.com . . . .
   . . . . .372, 161, 94, 260, 92, 124
aidsonline.com
   website of the medical

journal AIDS 372
alcohol 220
   and anti-HIV drugs 98
   and hepatitis 260
   health risks of heavy drinking . . .260
   safety of for people
   with hepatitis 221
   safety of for people
   with HIV 221, 260
   use of and increased risk of
   medication side-effects 221
Alcohol Concern 221
Alexander technique 202
allergic reaction 130
alpha-interferon 169
American Foundation for
AIDS Research (AMFAR) 373
amphetamines 222
   HIV disease progression faster
   amongst users of 222
amprenavir (*Agenerase*) 92
amylase .83
anabolic steroids 222, 269
   and the immune system 223
   as a treatment for lipodystrophy .138
   HIV transmission risk from
   needle sharing 223
anaemia 82, 172
anal cancer 37, 166
anal intraepithelial neoplasia 166
   personal experiences of 300
anal sex
   unprotected and hepatitis C
   transmission 169
anal sex, unprotected
   and HIV transmission 294
anomaly scan 190
anti-HIV drugs
   interractions with other medicines
   and drugs 98
   storage .99
anti-nausea medication 133
antidepressants 278, 276
antiretroviral therapy
   also see, HIV treatment 35
anxiety 274, 277
aromatherapy 201

asessingalanine
aminotransferase (ALT) 83
aspartate aminotransferase (AST) . . .83
asylum seekers
   benefits for 318
asymptomatic HIV infection 34
atazanavir (*Reyataz*) 92
atazanavir/ritonavir
   use in first-line treatment 93
attendance Allowance 314
autogenic training 202
autonomic neuropathy 142
AVERT 373
AZT (zidovudine, *Retrovir*) 191, 91
   as a cause of anaemia 83
   as a cause of lipodystrophy 135
   as a cause of nausea 133
   interaction with ribavirin 172
   monotherapy, personal
   experiences of 110
   side-effects 94
   use of to prevent dementia 274
   use of to prevent mother-to-baby
   transmission of HIV . .189, 190, 189

B

bach flower remedies 202
bacteria .161
barbiturates 223
bartonella (cat scratch disease) 211
beans 258
benefits .310
bilirubin .83
blackouts 160
bleach
   use of to clean injecting equipment . .
  237
bleeding disorders
   and resistance training 268
blood counts 82
boiling method
   to clean injecting equipment 237
breastfeeding
   and risk of mother-to-baby
   transmission of HIV 191

bronchitis 157
bronchoscopy 157
bupropion (*Zyban*) 235

C

caesarean delivery 190
   to reduce risk of mother-to-baby
   transmission of HIV 188
calcium supplements 262
campylobacter 214
cancer 161, 163, 166
cancers
   non-AIDS defining increase since
   introduction of HAART 166
candidiasis (thrush) 161
cannabis .223
   and pain relief 224
   as an appetite stimulant 224
   risks of using 224
carers 242
Carers Allowance 314
CD4 cell count 88, 74, 35, 34, 19
   and decision to start treatment . . .81
   and HIV infection 75
   and HIV treatment decisions 76
   and infections 74
   and methamphetamine use 227
   and smoking smoking 234
   frequency of monitoring 82
   increase after starting HIV
   treatment, personal
   experiences of 109
   low and risk of infections 156
   low and use of anti-HIV drugs to
   prevent mother-to-baby
   transmission of HIV 189
   low and vulnerability to infections . . .
  159
   lower in HIV-positive people
   who have unprotected sex 217
   normal ranges 74
   percentages 76
   regular monitoring 74
CD4 cells .32

   white blood cells 74
CD4 count, viral load
   and disease progression 81, 74
cervical cancer 167
chemotherapy 163
   for anal cancer 166
   for liver cancer 170
chest pain
   as a symptom of tuberculosis 165
chest problems 157
chest x-ray 157
chickenpox 210
Child Benefit 317
Child Tax Credit 317
children's hospitals
   and HIV treatment 58
cholesterol 139
   and anabolic steroid use 223
   exercise and 266
   personal experiences of changing
   HIV treatment because of 113
cholesterol tests 83
Cialis 228, 233
   and poppers 233
Citizens Advice Bureau . . .248, 67, 310
civil partnerships 322, 248, 247
   effect on state benefits 318
Clinical Care Options for HIV
   website 373
clinical trials
   into the treatment of primary
   HIV infection 89
co-trimoxazole 165
cocaine 225
cognitive behavioural therapy 278
cognitive behavioural therapy (CBT) . . .
  292
colds
   people with HIV, vulnerability to . . . .
  210
colds and flu 156
Combivir .92
   personal experiences of 109
community nurses 243
complaining about services 59
complementary and alternative therapies
   and stopping smoking 235
complementary therapies 198

A - Z of 201
and HIV treatment 200
choosing a practitioner 199
personal experiences of 110, 206
points to remember 199
reasons for use 198
use of to relieve emotional distress ..
........................276
concentration 160
condoms 356, 295
confidentiality 352
maintaining whilst in hospital ...246
confusion 160
constipation 159
constitutional symptoms 156
contraception
emergency 295
cosmetic surgery 103
cough
as a symptom of tuberculosis 165
coughs
risk from air travel 215
council services
to support independent living 242
council tax benefit 312
counselling
personal experiences of 27
post HIV-diagnosis 18
crack 225
cryptococcal meningitis 161
cryptosporidiosis 162
cryptosporidium 215, 211
crystal meth 227
cytomegalovirus (CMV) 144, 161
and eye problems 159

D

d4T (stavudine, *Zerit*) 91
and fat loss 102
as a cause of lipodystrophy 135
as a cause of nausea 133
as a cause of neuropathy 142
as a cause of sexual dysfunction .292
concerns about side-effects 93

interaction with ribavirin 172
use of to prevent dementia 274
DART study
termination 106
dairy produce 258
dapsone
as a cause of neuropathy 143
ddI (didanosine, *Videx/Videx EC*) ...91
as a cause of neuropathy 142
interaction with ribavirin 172
as a cause of sexual dysfunction .292
death 247
debt 248
decisions
about disclosure and treatment
post-diagnosis 19
dementia 162, 160, 274
dental health 64
dental hygiene 158
dentists 64
at HIV clinics 64
NHS 64
depression 37, 160, 276, 274
caused by efavirenz (*Sustiva*) ...277
diarrhoea 162, 159, 156, 211, 163
and diet 261
personal experiences of 7, 108
replacing lost nutrients 262
travelers 216
Dica, Mohammed
conviction for transmission of HIV ..
........................355
diet 258
dietary therapies 202
dietitians 269, 162, 258, 261
digestion problems 159
DIPEx 374
Disability Benefits Centre 314
Disability Discrimination Act ....
...............349, 360, 348, 47
Disability Living Allowance ...312, 311
disclosing HIV status 267
to a partner 45
to a sexual partner, personal
experience of 301
to children 49
to complementary health

practitioners 49
to dentists 47
to employers 46
to ex-sexual partners 45
to family 46
to friends 46
to GPs .47
to pharmacists 48
to sexual partners 45
disclosing HIV status to friends
personal experiences of 183
disclosure of confidential medical
information 353
disclosure of HIV status 44
at work .348
legal duty to disclose to sexual
partners 357
personal experiences of 8
practicalities 44
to partner, personal experiences of . . .
. 51
discrimination
personal experiences of 176
discrimination because of HIV
personal experiences of 22
Drinkline 221
driving
need for caution if medication
causes drowziness 100
drug companies
treatment information 100
drug dependency units
and HIV treatment 58
drug names
trade name and generic name 95
drug overdose 237
drug resistant HIV
transmission of 297
drug use .219
and the law 219

E

early doses 121
Easy Travel Insurance 339

eating
and exercise 269
ecstasy 228
risks of using 229
efavirenz (Sustiva) 92
as a cause of psychological
disturbances 277
dizziness 131
personal experiences of 109
use of to prevent dementia 274
eggs 258
emergencies
arrangements at HIV clinics 59
emergency medical treatment 156
emigration
and HIV 327
emotional distress 274, 275
emphysema
increased risk of in HIV-positive
smokers 234
Enhanced Disability Premium 313
entitlement to free NHS care 63
erythromycin 292
EU
entitlement to medical care within
when traveling 339
traveling within 326
European Economic Area
and immigration and asylum law .358
European Health Insurance Card . . . . .
. . . . .339, 65
exercise .202
benefits of 266
personal experiences of 205, 270
setting goals 266
exercise programmes 268
eye tests .159
eyes 159

F

facial wasting
d4T and AZT as a cause 136
vulnerability to if immune
system weak 132

fats

in diet 258
fever

as a symptom of tuberculosis 165
fevers 156, 163
fibrates 102, 141
finances

after a death 248

sorting out before death 247
fish 258
fish oil 261, 142
fisting

hepatitis C virus transmission . . .169
fluids

intake and exercise 268
fluoxetine (Prozac)

as a cause of sexual dysfunction .291
food

safety .215
food poisoning 214
food restrictions

and adherence 98
formula feed

to prevent mother-to-baby
transmission of HIV 191
formula feeding

to reduce risk of mother-to-baby
transmission of HIV 188
fosamprenavir (Telzir) 92
fosamprenavir/ritonavir

use in first-line treatment 93
Freedom Travel Insurance 339
fruit 258
fruit juice

safety of 213
FTC (emtricitabine, Emtriva) 92

treatment for hepatitis B 94

treatment for hepatitis B virus . .168
funeral arrangements 248
funerals .247
fungi 161

fusion inhibitor 92

G

gardening

hygiene precautions 211
garlic

interaction with HIV treatment . .199

interaction with HIV treatments .259
gay men

personal experiences of treatment . . .
. 145

HIV-positive and sexual transmission
of hepatitis C virus 169
genital warts

personal experiences of 299
GHB (gammahydroxybutyrate) 230
glitazones 142
glucose 140
glucose test 83
GMFA 370
GP

personal experiences of using 22
GPs 242, 61

importance of 61
GUM clinics

and HIV treatment 58

H

HAART
(highly active antiretroviral therapy)

also see, HIV treatment 36
haematology units

and HIV treatment 58
haemophilia 268

infection with hepatitis C virus . .169

personal experiences of 180
head problems 159
headache .159
health advisers 294
Health Protection Agency 295
heart disease 140

HIV-positive smokers and risk of . . . .
. 234

personal experiences of 7
heart disease and anti-HIV drugs . .141

heart rate
  and exercise 266
helplines 21
hepatitis A virus
  and alcohol 260
  vaccination 216
hepatitis B virus 293, 167, 37
  and alcohol 260
  coinfection in people with HIV . . . . .
    .167, 166
  HIV disease progression 168
  testing 168
  treatment 168
  vaccination 216, 168
hepatitis B virus and HIV coinfection
  UK treatment guidelines 169
Hepatitis C Information Line 369
hepatitis C virus 37, 293
  aims of treatment 172
  and alcohol 260
  and HIV disease progression 171
  as a cause of liver cancer 170
  coinfection in people with HIV . . . . .
    .166, 167
  factors involved in disease
  progression 170
  genotype 171
  mother-to-baby transmission 169
  natural history 170
  personal experiences of 180
  sexual transmission of 169
  side-effects of treatment 172
  symptoms 169
  testing 170
  transmission 169
  treatment 171
hepatitis C virus and HIV coinfection
  treatment strategies 172
  UK treatment guidelines 172
hepatitis C virus viral load test (PCR) . .
   170
herbal remedies 259, 202
  interaction with HIV drugs 118
heroin 230
herpes simplex virus 158, 159

herpes simplex virus-2 293
high blood pressure
  HIV-positive smokers and risk of . . . .
   234
HIV 32
  and complementary therapies . . .198
  and confidentiality 352
  and hepatitis C virus disease
  progression 170
  and smoking 234
  antibodies to 33
  as a cause of mental health problems
   274
  as a continuing cause of death . . .247
  as a continuing cause of illness
  and death 242
  blood-to-blood transmission of 33
  disease progression and cocaine use . .
   226
  disease progression and
  methamphetamine use 227
  disease progression and opiates . .232
  dismissal from work because of . .349
  HIV disease progression and
  use of ecstasy 228
  illness due to, personal
  experiences of 178
  mother-to-child transmission of . . .33
  no cure .88
  personal experiences of . . . .
    . . . . .12, 283, 40, 282, 39, 180, 284
  reinfection with drug resistant HIV . .
   216
  replication in the brain and organs 88
  risk of illness increases longer there is
  no treatment 34
  sexual transmission of 32
  superinfection with drug
  resistant HIV 216
  transmission of 32
  treatment 88
HIV antibody test 33
HIV clinics 19, 58
  access to dentists 59
  access to mental health specialists . . .
   59

availability of mental health teams 276
better survival at larger ones 60
HIV diagnosis 18
and feelings about sex 290
personal experiences of ....
...112, 270, 22, 108, 26, 10, 24, 23
HIV disease progression
and use of complementary therapies .
........................198
personal experiences of 108
HIV doctors
relationship with 60
specialists 60
HIV encephalopathy 162
HIV testing
at work 348
HIV transmission as a crime ....
...................355 293, 216
effect of consent 356
legal duty to disclose HIV status .357
use of condoms 356
HIV treatment 80
aim of in people with lots of
treatment experience 88
and cannabis use 225
and cocaine use 226
and complementary therapies ...200
and diet 260
and digestive problems 159
and head problems 159
and hepatitis C coinfection 90
and interaction with bupropion
(Zyban) 235
and interaction with ecstasy 229
as a cause of mental
health problems 274
availability throughout the UK 58
changing because of side-effects,
personal experiences of 148
changing due to failure 101
changing due to side-effects 101
during primary infection 89, 34
effective treatment for Kaposi's
sarcoma 163

if no symptoms of HIV 90
if there are symptoms of HIV 90
if you have drug resistant HIV ..103
illnesses rarer because of 160
improvement in prognosis for
people with HIV 165
inability to eradicate HIV from
the body 88
interaction with methadone 231
limited impact of changing on
body shape changes 103
lymphoma rarer because of 163
personal experiences of .114, 38, 147
poppers, interaction with 233
resistance, personal experiences of .11
safety for people coinfected with
hepatitis C virus 171
safety of to prevent mother-to-baby
transmission of HIV 190
side-effects, personal experiences of ..
..........................11
smokers at higher risk of increased
blood fats as a side-effect 234
starting, personal experiences of ....
...............112, 108, 107, 11
to prevent mother-to-baby
transmission of HIV 188, 190
travelling with 338
UK guidelines 89
use of in babies to prevent
mother-to-baby transmission
of HIV 190
when to start 88
HIV treatment interruption
personal experiences of 11
HIVandHepatitis.com 373
HIVInsite.com 373
holidays
problems which anti-HIV drugs
can cause 99
holidays and medication
personal experiences of 341
homoeopathy 203
hospital
admission to 243

admission to for reasons other
than HIV 60
discharge from 246
going into, personal experiences of . . .
. 253
making more comfortable 245
visitors whilst admitted to 244
hospital appointments
time off work for 348
Housing benefit 312
human growth hormone
as a treatment for lipodystrophy .138
human papilloma virus (HPV) 166
hygiene 210
hypnotherapy 203
and stopping smoking 235
hypogonadism 292

I

i-Base Treatment Phoneline 369
ibuprofen 160, 165
illness
coping with 242
personal experiences of .38, 175, 177
immigration and asylum law 357
entering UK for medical treatment359
entry to UK if HIV-positive 358
HIV as grounds to remain in the UK .
. 359
the relevance of being HIV-positive ..
. 358
Immigration and Nationality Directorate
. 67
Immigration Law Practitioners
Association 67
immigration restrictions for people
with HIV 326
immune system 32
use of complementary therapies to
boost 198
immunisations 216
live 216
imodium .262
Incapacity Benefit 310

Income Support 311
independent living 242
indinavir (Crixivan) 92
and cannabis use 225
as a cause of anaemia 83
as a cause of nausea 133
levels of and large doses of
vitamin C 259
need for kidney function tests
if taking .84
infections
use of complementary therapies
to treat .199
injecting
safer 235
injecting equipment
cleaning 236
safe disposal of 237
inpatient care for people with HIV . .59
insulin 140
International AIDS Society (IAS) . .373
international travel 215
precautions 215
isoniazid
as a cause of neuropathy 143
itraconazole (Sporanox) 292

J

Job Seekers Allowance 315
Joint Council for the Welfare of
Immigrants 67

K

Kaletra (lopinavir/ritonavir)
use in first-line treatment 93
Kaposi's sarcoma 166, 162
no evidence that caused by poppers233
Kaposi's sarcoma treatment
side-effects of 143

Kelly, Stephen
    conviction for transmission of HIV ..
   355
ketamine 230
ketoconazole (*Nizoral*) 292
kidney function test 84
kidney stones
    and indinavir (*Crixivan*) 269
Kivexa 92

L

L-Acetyl-Carnitine
    as a treatment for peripheral
    neuropathy 143
lactic acidosis 131, 172
    Test for 83
late doses 121
life assurance 322
lipodystrophy 102, 131, 134
    and diet 261
    avoiding 136
    benefits of exercise for 266
    changing treatment to avoid 137
    emotional impact of 103
    living with body fat changes 139
    metabolic changes 139, 135
    patterns of body fat change 134
    personal experiences of ....
    ....145, 150, 7, 11
    risk of 135
    stopping treatment to avoid 137
    symptoms of metabolic change ..140
    treating fat gain 138
    treating fat loss 138
lipomas 135
listeria 214
liver biopsies 170
liver cancer 167
    treatment 170
liver cirrhosis 170
liver damage
    and inappropriate use of
    anabolic steroids 269
liver fibrosis 170

liver function
    effect of HIV drugs on 169
liver function tests 83, 168, 170
    and detection of hepatitis B or
    hepatitis C infection 83
liver transplants 172
liver, the 167
living wills 247
lopinavir/ritonavir (*Kaletra*) 92
LSD 231
lung cancer 37, 235, 167
lymphoma 160, 163

M

MAI 163
managed vaginal birth
    circumstances where safe 191
massage 203
meat........................258
medical retirement 322
Medicines Act 219
Medscape 374
memory loss 160
meningitis 160
Mens rea 356
mental health 274
    personal experiences of 6
metabolic tests 83
metformin 142
    as a treatment for lipodystrophy .138
methadone
    interaction with HIV medication .231
methamphetamine 227
Misuse of Drugs Act 219
mitochondrial toxicity
    personal experiences of 110
money 310
money worries
    personal experiences of 8
mortgages 322
Motability....................314
mother-to-baby transmission of HIV ...
   188
mouth ulcers 159
mulloscum 158

N

National Drugs Helpline 368
National Sexual Health Helpline ......
.....................368, 21
Nationality, Immigration and
Asylum Act 2002 357
naturopathy 203
nausea 159
   as a side-effect of HIV treatment ...
.......................133
   coping with 133
   personal experiences of 108
NAZ Project..................370
needle exchanges 236
nelfinavir (Viracept) 92, 262
neuropathy 142
   as a side-effect of anti-HIV drugs ...
.......................142
nevirapine (Viramune) 296, 92
   as a cause of liver toxicity 83
   cautions about use of to prevent
   mother-to-baby transmission of HIV .
.......................189
   use of to prevent mother-to-baby
   transmission of HIV 190, 189
New Fill 138, 103
NHS
   free HIV care 58
   free sexual health treatment 294
NHS care and EEA nationals 65
NHS care and non-UK nationals 64
NHS Direct 368, 63
nicotine replacement therapy 235
night sweats 156, 163
non-Hodgkins lymphoma 166
non-nucleoside reverse transcriptase
inhibitors (NNRTIs) 92
   and sexual dysfunction drugs 234
   based treatment 92
   metabolisation of 121
NucleomaxX 139
nucleoside analogue reverse
transcriptase inhibitors (NRTIs) .93, 91
nucleoside/nucleotide analogues
   side-effects 94
nucleotide analogue reverse
transcriptase inhibitors (NtRTIs) ...92

nurse-led clinics
   sexual health and adherence 59
nutrition
   personal experiences of 205
nuts 258

O

oat bran tablets
   as a diarrhoea treatment 262
occupational therapists 243
opiates 231
   use of and health risks of 231
opportunistic infections 32, 210
   risk of developing 74
oral hairy leukoplakia 159
oral sex 295
oral thrush 158
   risk of and smoking 234
osteopathy 203
outreach
   needle exchanges 236

P

pain
   treatment for 143
pain control
   advice from HIV clinics 243
pain relief
   use of complementary therapies for ..
.......................199
palliative care 243
pancreatitis 172, 83
PAP smears
   screening for anal cancer 166
   screening for cervical cancer 167
paracetamol 160, 156
paroxetine (Seroxat)
   as a cause of sexual dysfunction .291
partner
   death, personal experiences of ...250
   illness, personal experiences of ..250

PCP
   risk of and smoking 234
PCP pneumonia . . . .
. . .157, 74, 35, 76, 163, 166, 160, 165
pegylated interferon 172
pension
   beneficiaries 248
pensions 322
pentamidine
   as a cause of neuropathy 143
peripheral neuropathy 160, 142
   personal experiences of . . . .
   . . . . .146, 7, 147, 149
   vitamin B6 as a cause of 259
   vulnerability to if immune
   system weak 132
persistent generalised lymphadenopathy
   see, swollen glands 34
personal finance 310
pets 210
pharmacies
   and needle exchanges 236
pharmacists
   as a source of treatment information .
  100
   specialist HIV 59
physiotherapists 243
platelets .164
poppers 228, 232
Positive Nation Magazine 371
Positively Women 371
post-exposure prophylaxis (PEP) . .296
poultry 258
Power of Attorney 248
pregnancy .99
   personal experiences of HIV
   diagnosis during 192
pregnancy and HIV
   personal experiences of 193
prognosis 247
   for people with HIV 36
   personal expectations of 24
property
   inheritance of 248
prophylaxis 161
   for opportunistic infections 35
   PCP 164

protease inhibitors 92
   and blood fats 102
   and sexual dysfunction drugs 234
   as a cause of liver toxicity 83
   as a cause of sexual dysfunction .292
   based treatment 93
   boosted by ritonavir 93
   metabolisation of 121
   resistannce to, personal
   experiences of 110
protozoa and parasites 161
psychotherapy 278

Q

Quitline 235

R

radiotherapy 163
   for anal cancer 166
reckless endangerment 357
recreational drug use and anti-HIV
medication
   personal experiences of 206
recreational drugs
   interaction with HIV drugs 118
red blood cells 157
   and zinc 259
reflexology 203
Refugee Legal Centre 67
reinfection 297, 293
rented property
   succession to tenancy 248
resistance .80
   and NNRTIs 93
   as a result of poor adherence . . .118
   cross-resistance between drugs . .118
   difficulty of getting an undetectable
   viral load due to 103
   risk of if stop treatment beacuse of
   lipodystrophy 137

resistance test

personal experiences of 111

resistance tests 101, 104

before starting HIV treatment 91

resistance training 267

and cholesterol 266

retroviruses 32

ribavirin .172

interaction with HIV drugs 172

right of abode in UK 358

ritonavir (*Norvir*) 92

and interaction with ecstasy 229

and methamphetamine use 228

as a cause of nausea 133

full dose, interaction with erectile

dysfunction drugs 292

S

safer sex .216

salmonella 214

salvage therapy 104

personal experiences of 145

saquinavir (hard gel, Invirase) 92

saquinavir/ritonavir

use in first-line treatment 93

schizophrenia 162

seborrhoeic dermatitis 158

selective serotonin re-uptake

inhibitors (SSRIs) 276

selenium .259

seroconversion illness 33

symptoms of 33

serum albumin 83

Severe Disability Premium 313

Severe Disablement Allowance 312

sex 290

unprotected, as risk factor for faster

HIV disease progression 216

sexual dysfunction 291

sexual dysfunction drugs 233

sexual health 293

sexual health check-ups 293

sexual health clinics 293

sexual problems

as a treatment side-effect 130

post HIV-diagnosis, personal

experiences of 50

sexually transmitted infections . . . .

. . . . .216, 293

and HIV transmission 295

transmission as a potential criminal

offence 355

shaitsu 204

Shigella .214

sick leave 348

side-effects 130, 165, 156

and NNRTIs 93

and peak drug leves 131

as a reason for treatment change 102

chaning HIV treatment because of

. 132

daily pattern of 131

head problems 160

identifying the cause 132

longer term 131

medicines to control 132, 131

personal experiences of 7, 108

questions about when starting

anti-HIV treatment 95

relief of .96

stopping or interruption

treatment because of 97

timing of after starting anti-HIV

treatment 96

types of 130

use of complementary therapies

to reduce 198

vulnerability to if immune

system weak 132

weighing up risk of against benefits

of treatment 132

when they occur 131

sildenafil (*Viagra*) 292

skin problems 158

sleep

problems caused by efavirenz

(*Sustiva*) 277

SMART study

termination 106

smoking 234
    as a risk factor for disease progression
    if infected with hepatitis B or C
    viruses .170
Social Fund, the 321, 320
speech problems 160
sputum culture 157
St Johns wort
    interaction with HIV treatment . . . . .
    . . . . .199, 49
    interaction with protease inhibitors
    and NNRTIs 276
starchy food 258
statins 102, 141
    as a treatment for fat loss 139
Statutory Maternity Allowance 317
Statutory Maternity Pay 316
Statutory Sick Pay 310
stopping smoking 235
stopping treatment
    because of peripheral neuropathy . . . .
   143
stress
    use of complementary therapies
    to reduce 198
structured treatment interruptions . .105
    personal experiences of 110
students
    benefits for 318
studying .347
suicidal impulse 162
sulphonylureas 142
supplements 259
    and HIV treatment 200
support groups
    for people who have been
    recently diagnosed 21
surgery
    for anal cancer 166
    for liver cancer 170
swallowing
    pain and difficulty 159
swimming
    risk of water-borne infections . . .214
swollen glands
    as a symptom of HIV infection . . .34

syphilis
    routine testing for as part of HIV care
   84

T

T-20 (enfuvirtide, *Fuzeon*) 92
    when to use 104
T-cell chronicles 374
T-cells 74
tadalafil (Cialis) 292
tai chi 202
temperature 157
tenofovir (Viread) 92
    interaction with ribavirin 172
    switch to as a treatment for fat loss .
   137
    treatment for hepatitis B 94
    treatment for hepatitis B virus . .168
    use in initial HIV treatment regimens
   94
Terrence Higgins Trust 369
testicular cancer 37, 167
testosterone replacement therapy . .222
The Body
    website 374
therapeutic touch 202
thrombocytopenia 164
THT Direct 21, 369, 310
tipranavir (*Aptivus*) 92
tiredness 156
TMC114 105
tobacco 234
toxoplasmosis 160, 210, 165
traditional Chinese medicine 204
training 346
travel 326
    and adherence 338
    and health 339
    and treatment breaks 340
travel insurance 339, 215, 326
treatment breaks
    and travel 340
triglycerides 140
    exercise and 266
Trizivir 92

trol acetate (*Megace*)

as a cause of sexual dysfunction .292
Truvada 92
tuberculosis 166, 165, 163, 160

and starting HIV treatment 91

BCG vaccination 216

multi-drug resistant 165

personal experiences of 178

U

UK Coalition of People Living with HIV
and AIDS (UKC) 59, 371
ultrasound examinations 170, 168
UNAIDS 374
undetectable viral load 78, 79

as an aim of HIV treatment ..88, 81

desirability of 80
unprotected sex

and sexual dysfunction drugs 233

poppers as a trigger for 233
USA

and entry restrictions for people with

HIV 326

V

vaccinations

and travel 340

for travel 326
vaginal sex, unprotected

and HIV transmission 294
valium 158
vardenafil (Levitra) 292
vegetables 258
Viagra 233, 228

and poppers 233
viral load 78

and HIV transmission 295

blips 80

in women 80

rebound 88
reducing, aim of HIV treatment ...88
regular monitoring 74
relationship with CD4 cell count ..78
undetectable and infectiousness ..297
undetectable, personal experiences of .
.....................110, 109
viral load tests ...33, 78, 74, 35, 34, 19

and subtypes of HIV 78

before starting treatment 82

blips 101

effect of vaccinations 79

fluctuation 79

frequency of monitoring 82

HIV RNA 78

PCR 78

to monitor effectiveness of

treatment 81

unltrasensitive 78
virus 161
visualisation 204
vitamin A 259
vitamin B-12 144
vitamin B6 259
vitamin C 259

interaction with HIV treatment ..199
vitamins 259
voluntary services

to support independent living 242
volunteering 346

W

warts 158

personal experiences of 8
washing-up liquid

use of to clean injecting equipment 237
water

drinking, safety of 211

filters 212

mineral, safety of 212

overseas, safety of 213

weight loss 159, 261
   as a symptom of tuberculosis 165
   white blood cells
   and zinc 259
wills 247
work
   help returning to 347
   returning to 346
Working Tax Credit 315

Y

yoga 202

Z

zinc 259